MW01014203

Excess Face Height Malocclusion:

Etiology, Diagnosis, and Treatment

Excess Face Height Malocclusion:

Etiology, Diagnosis, and Treatment

Sten Linder-Aronson, DDS, PhD, PhD (hc)

Professor
Department of Orthodontics
Karolinska Institutet, Stockholm, Sweden

University of Athens, Greece
University of Sun-Yat-Sen, Guangzhou, China

Donald G. Woodside, CM, DDS, MSc, PhD (hc), FRCD(Can), FDSRCS (Eng)

Professor
Discipline of Orthodontics
University of Toronto, Toronto, Canada

Karolinska Institutet, Stockholm, Sweden

quintessence books

Quintessence Publishing Co, Inc

Chicago, Berlin, London, Tokyo, Paris, Barcelona,
São Paulo, Moscow, Prague, and Warsaw

Library of Congress Cataloging-in-Publication Data

Linder-Aronson, Sten, 1930–
    Excess face height malocclusion: etiology, diagnosis, and treatment / Sten
Linder-Aronson, Donald G. Woodside
        p.   ;   cm.
    Includes bibliographical references and index.
    ISBN 0-86715-389-X
    1. Malocclusion. 2. Face—Growth. 3. Cephalometry. I. Woodside, Donald G. II. Title.
    [DNLM: 1. Malocclusion—etiology. 2. Cephalometry. 3. Face—anatomy & histology.
    4. Mouth Breathing—complications. 5. Nasal Obstruction—complications. 6. Vertical
    Dimension. WU 440 L744e 2000]
    RK523 .L565 2000
    617.5'2—dc21

                                                                    00-027818

quintessence
books

© 2000 Quintessence Publishing Co, Inc

Quintessence Publishing Co, Inc
551 Kimberly Drive
Carol Stream, Illinois 60188

Editor: Paul Engman
Design/Production: Mike Shanahan/Sue Robinson

Printed in the USA

Dedication

The authors would like to express our deep thanks and love to our wives, Margareta and Sheila, for their devotion during the long hours spent in writing this book. We would also like to dedicate this volume to our dear colleague, Dr T.M. Graber, who has supported our orthodontic careers so graciously through many years.

Contents

Foreword

Some of the most challenging and deforming malocclusions facing the orthodontist are vertical problems. For too long, clinicians have concentrated on sagittal problems, with an assist from transverse mechanotherapy. In so doing, their efforts have often exacerbated the long face symptomatology, enhancing functional and esthetic compensations. The landmark studies of Professors Linder-Aronson and Woodside have been the best source of information on etiology, diagnosis, and treatment of these difficult malocclusions with their skeletal and neuromuscular malrelationships. Their long-term assessment of the effect of removal of excessive epipharyngeal tissue clearly shows the multisystem relationships of hard and soft tissues and compensatory functional exacerbations.

This monograph "puts it all together" for both scientists and clinicians as we enter the new millennium. Materia technica development has been superb, but what about the biophysiological considerations? Harry Sicher, the great anatomist, said it so well: "Whenever there is a struggle be-

tween muscle and bone, bone yields!" A study of orthodontic history shows the ebb and flow of expansionist treatment philosophies as orthodontists are mesmerized by efficient mechanical tooth-moving appliances with glowing commercial claims and selected case reports. Currently, the expansionist school dominates the "tooth straighteners," who have the efficient mechanotherapy to readily produce tooth positional changes. Along with this is the retention philosophy of "holding them forever." The twin scourges of iatrogenic damage and lack of stability after appliance removal remain. This is ever more apparent with our improved means of assessing changes by more sophisticated, long-term, diagnostic tools and the concerns expressed by periodontists and in the research, literature, and courts. Does it have to be "What price orthodontics?" Can we not accept the challenge of the new century and become true applied biologists?

This volume is a major step in the right direction by two world-class clinicians and researchers. The eight chapters give the biological background and supportive research to better understand the relationship between skeletal dysplasias and nasopharyngeal morphology.

Chapter 1 supports the view that environmental and neuromuscular influences may alter facial and dental structures. Elimination of deleterious factors may allow some recovery of these dysplasias. Nasopharyngeal and oropharyngeal obstructions are major concerns, but other multiple factors are discussed, ie, allergic rhinitis, sleep apnea, deviated septum, choanal atresia, altered mandibular posture, altered tongue posture and function, head posture, incorrect orthodontic treatment, thumb sucking, deglutition, etc. These conditions may exist in combination, of course, enhancing or offsetting their effect on growth and development. The creation of excessive face height by neuromuscular factors is not meant to imply that this is the only factor involved, although it may have been the most neglected one. Morphogenetic pattern is still a major consideration. Diagnosis is the name of the game–and early!

Dentofacial changes associated with chronic mandibular posture change, with and without mouth breathing, are discussed. Pertinent studies support the succinct discussion.

Reversal of symptoms following adenoidectomy and change of breathing mode are graphically illustrated. Studies are cited to support and to question some of the conclusions. Change in growth direction is another factor that has an impact on the ultimate dentofa-

cial morphology and supportive research substantiates the discussion by the authors. Specific effects on tooth position of neuromuscular aberrations and their elimination are shown, an excellent example of applied biology. Those who adhere to nonextraction, expansionist mechanotherapy would do well to read this research-supported discussion.

Chapter 2 presents three samples of pertinent studies from the Burlington Growth Centre, the Örebro adenoid study, and the King's College School of Medicine and Dentistry growth study. These are landmark contributions to the field and have broad application to all craniofacial growth studies.

Chapter 3 describes radiographic techniques, enlargements, and measurements for both the lateral cephalogram and the 45-degree oblique view. Landmarks and measurements are presented. Research methodology must be rigorous and readily duplicated by other researchers.

Chapter 4 gives population standards for mandibular growth (distance curves), which serve as a basis for determination of departure from norms. These provide a biological yardstick for both clinicians and researchers. When does natural variation become abnormal?

Chapter 5 is an interesting comparison of standards from various growth centers and for different races. Five different studies provide a basis for Caucasian, Asian, and African-American assessment. Appropriately, we are one world of orthodontics!

Chapter 6 records the nasal resistance standards, again giving the clinician a basis of what to expect in a normal sample. This is important to the otologist and pediatrician as well as to the orthodontist. Visual inspection of nasal structures alone is not adequate. This compilation of data should serve as a springboard for further studies of the age-linked role of respiration in dentofacial growth and development.

Chapter 7 is a fascinating tour de force for the orthodontist, rhinologist, pediatrician, and associated disciplines in the discussion of clinical applications of vertical changes in the jaws and dentition. Cephalometric identification of the true nature of skeletal dysplasias and an analysis of anteroposterior nasopharyngeal dimension are elaborated for both the clinical and research viewpoint. On the basis of these studies, the skeletal pattern is not immutable, but subject to some modification.

Chapter 8 is a succinct summary. Together with Chapter 1, the reader gets a concise but comprehensive appraisal of the dynamic role of hard and soft tissue interaction. The excellent illustrations throughout the volume provide more than ample validation for the concepts presented. As the authors state so well in the Preface, "The neuromuscular suspension of the mandible is a highly sensitive mechanism that responds with altered mandibular posture in some cases of chronic nasopharyngeal obstruction." Surely, as this monograph demonstrates so well, differential diagnosis and treatment timing are of paramount importance.

For readers stimulated by the monograph, an excellent up-to-date bibliography provides excellent coverage of the field and ample basis for continuing research. The authors are to be congratulated for this superb contribution to our compendium of knowledge.

Thomas M. Graber, DMD, MSD, PhD
Chicago, Illinois

Preface

The motive in undertaking this book is to present the results of 30 years of research on the effect of environmental factors on craniofacial growth. The relationship between nasal obstruction and altered facial and dental structures has been discussed for at least 150 years and conflicting opinions have been presented. The authors therefore believed it important to gather their results from years of carefully controlled studies to clarify the controversy over this relationship.

During the 19th century and to the middle of the 20th, the ideas concerning the relationship between mouth breathing and malocclusion were based on clinical observation and experience. After cephalometric longitudinal material became available in the latter part of the 20th century, it was possible to obtain research results from controlled studies. It has also become possible during the past few decades to measure airflow through the nose and nasal resistance in accurate ways, which thus enabled statistical analyses.

Study of the vertical dimensions of the face in relation to the mode of breathing and to the posture of both the head and the mandible provides an excellent model to support the view that many malocclusions previously thought to be of genetic origin are in reality neuromuscular imitations of genetically based problems. The neuromuscular suspension of the mandible is a highly sensitive mechanism that responds with altered mandibular posture in some cases of chronic nasopharyngeal obstruction. Such altered mandibular posture may create various malocclusions in children.

The results gathered in this book are based on scientific longitudinal materials from the Burlington Growth Centre in Toronto, Canada, and Swedish adenoid samples from Stockholm and Örebro. Comparisons are made with longitudinal cephalometric materials from growth centers in Europe, North America, and Asia. The evaluations of the capacity to breathe through the mouth and/or the nose were made in collaboration with the ear, nose, and throat departments at the Hospital for Sick Children in Toronto, Canada, and at the University of Örebro, Sweden, by using both rhinomanometric and clinical tools.

This book is designed to be used by both dental and medical students in the specialized areas of orthodontics and rhinology. It will also be of great interest for clinical orthodontists, ear, nose, and throat specialists, and pediatricians.

The authors would like to acknowledge the contribution of the staff of the Burlington Growth Centre, who worked for so many years under the able direction of the late Dr F. Popovich. Their devotion and energy were responsible for the collection and maintenance of much of the material used in the preparation of this book. We would also like to acknowledge the contribution of Dr Robert Moyers, who had the foresight and imagination to initiate the Burlington Growth Centre Study. We are further indebted to Dr Egil Harvold and Dr Margaret Hatton for the continuation of the Centre during difficult times.

We thank Professor Emeritus Barry Leighton of King's College School of Medicine and Dentistry in London, England, for access to data from the longitudinal sample that he collected for 40 years. Our deep thanks to Caroline Chu and Joanne Hofmeister, who typed the manuscript.

Factors Affecting Facial and Dental Structures

Evidence has accumulated during recent years that supports the view that environmental and neuromuscular influences may alter facial and dental structures. These morphologic changes may show some recovery following the removal of the deleterious impact. Harvold et al[39,41] concluded from their nonhuman primate experiments that any factor lowering the postural position of the mandible will promote additional tooth eruption and increased lower anterior face height. One such factor is an obstructed nasopharyngeal airway.[35]

Nasopharyngeal Obstruction

The nasopharynx is a vaultlike structure that extends from the base of the skull to the level of the hard palate. The choanae form the anterior border of the nose, whereas the pharyngeal isthmus forms the lower border toward the oropharynx. Adenoid hypertrophy is one common cause of nasopharyngeal obstruction. It is important for the orthodontist to know the growth pattern of the posterior nasopharyngeal wall when evaluating the nasopharyngeal airway on a lateral cephalogram. The relationship between the soft tissue pharyngeal thickness and the bony nasopharynx size determines the airway size and may influence the mode of breathing. The adenoids are small at birth due to the immature state of the immune system. The adenoids enlarge and eventually outstrip the growth of the nasopharyngeal space at 3 to 5 years, thereby reducing the nasopharyngeal airway size. However, after age 5, expansion of the bony nasopharyngeal space continues due to maxillary growth. Percentile distance curves for the amount of soft tissue and adenoids on the posterior nasopharyngeal wall show a peak at age 5 and 10 to 11 years. Thereafter, a steady decline in these tissues occurs as children mature.[55]

Oropharyngeal Obstruction

The oropharyngeal space is situated dorsal to the tongue. Obstruction of the oropharyngeal space can also be caused by grossly enlarged tonsils due to chronic or recurrent acute tonsillitis. Enlarged tonsils may lead to a forward displacement of the tongue and a caudal displacement of the hyoid bone, changes that are reversed after a tonsillectomy.[10] The following list of selected investigations has confirmed associations with malocclusions characterized by increased lower anterior face height.

1. Genetic predisposition[61]
2. Enlarged adenoids[50]
3. Enlarged tonsils[9]
4. Allergic rhinitis[105]
5. Sleep apnea[2,46]
6. Deviated nasal septum[30]
7. Choanal atresia[29]
8. Altered mandibular posture[35]
9. Altered tongue posture[35]
10. Extended head posture[79]
11. Incorrect orthodontic treatment, eg, creation of dual bite[40]
12. Amelogenesis imperfecta[70]
13. Weakness in the muscles of mastication[87]
14. Thumb-sucking[49]

It is apparent from this list that a number of interrelated factors may operate to produce the dentofacial changes which have been documented in chronic mouth-breathing cases. In all of these conditions, one or all of three neuromuscular responses must be present for malocclusion and altered skeletal relationships to occur. These are:

1. Altered mandibular posture. The mandible rotates down and back in response to the etiologic factor.
2. Altered tongue posture. The tongue moves superiorly and anteriorly in response to the etiologic factor.
3. Extended head posture. The mandible is held in position while the cranium and maxilla rotate upward.

Diagnostic factors such as nasopharyngeal obstruction and increased nasal resistance may be relatively unimportant in individuals. The important point is the individual's neuromuscular response to the initial stimulus. For example, if an individual with upper airway obstruction does not respond in one or all of the stated three ways, no malocclusion will ensue. Instead, the individual may respond by breathing with increased chest activity to overcome the obstruction. Whether air flows through the nose or the mouth is less important

Dentofacial Characteristics Associated with Chronic Change in Mandibular Posture

Much interest has been directed to the relationship between breathing patterns and vertical facial development in an attempt to clarify the operative basic biologic principles. One must first distinguish between nose and mouth breathers to be able to discuss respiratory function and its effect on tongue and mandibular posture. The problem arises in that individuals described as mouth breathers also retain some ability to breathe through the nose. Indeed, some grossly obstructed individuals continue to force air through the nose by using more effort in breathing.[71] On the other hand, some people with clear nasopharyngeal passages are habitual mouth breathers. As a general principle, most authorities consider that mouth breathing will become obligatory above a certain level of nasal resistance. However, only patients with total blockage of the nasal airway, such as bilateral choanal atresia or nasal alar insufficiency, may be described as pure mouth breathers. In all other cases, combinations of nasal and oral respiration are found. When we speak of mouth breathers, we are therefore referring to those individuals who have a certain capacity for nose breathing but, for one reason or another, breathe mainly through the mouth.

One group of patients who often have reduced nasal respiratory function are those with enlarged adenoid tissue. The dentofacial morphology of these patients can be studied following an adenoidectomy. They thus provide an excellent research model for examining the possible effects on dentofacial development of changes in the mode of breathing and subsequent alterations in tongue and mandibular posture. Such patients have been used as an experimental model to clarify basic biologic principles.

Linder-Aronson's landmark study[50] compared 81 children who had severe nasal obstruction and mouth-open breathing to an equal number of nose breathers with mouth-closed breathing. The two groups were matched for similar age and sex. The differences in facial morphology found between the two groups are seen in Fig 1-1. The children with obstructed nasal breathing were characterized by an increased lower face height, increased total facial height, and more retrognathic jaws compared with the control children. Further, the sagittal depth of the bony nasopharynx was small compared with the controls. The tongue position was also altered forward.

Figure 1-2 shows the typical facial morphology of a child with chronic nasal obstruction and associated mouth-open posture. The typical dentition of such children shows retroclined incisors in both arches, a narrow maxillary arch, a posterior crossbite, incisor crowding in both jaws, and, in some individuals, a tendency toward an anterior open bite. It has been suggested that these differences in facial and dental morphology could be due to differences in the underlying morphogenetic pattern. However, accumulating evidence shows that neuromuscular and environmental factors can also produce these symptoms in affected individuals. For example, the lower anterior facial height was com-

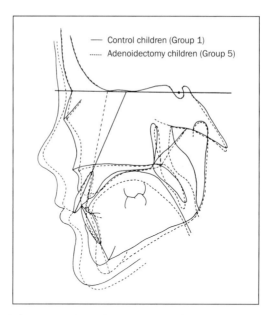

Fig 1-1 Tracings of lateral cephalometric radiographs showing significant mean differences between children who had adenoidectomy for obstructed nose breathing and the controls. The variables represent adenoids, the dentition, the skeleton, the lips, and tongue position.

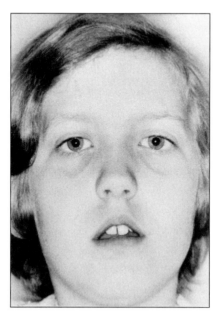

Fig 1-2 An individual who shows the typical facial characteristics of long-standing nasal obstruction and associated mouth breathing (adenoid facies).

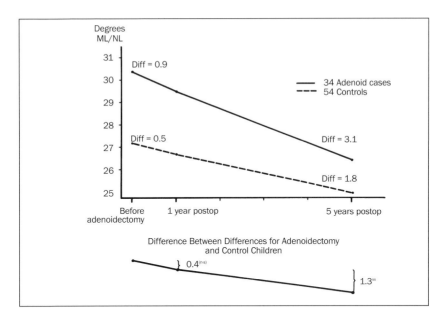

Fig 1-3 Changes in the angle between the mandibular plane (ML) and the palatal plane (NL) following a change from mouth to nose breathing over a 5-year period following adenoidectomy. During the first year postoperatively, there was no significant difference for mandibular plane flattening between controls and operated cases. During the following 4 years, the operated cases changed more than the matched controls (p < 0.01). In other words, a normalization of the lower face height occurred throughout the total observation period of 5 years between ages 7 and 12 years.

pared in a nasal obstruction group who had mouth-open posture to a nose-breathing group.[52] Comparisons were done preadenoidectomy and 1 and 5 years postadenoidectomy. The mean age of the children was initially 7.5 years. Following adenoidectomy, those children in the nasal obstruction group who changed their mode of breathing from mouth to nose breathing were selected for further study. Figure 1-3 shows how the lower anterior face height improved in these children. During the total 5-year observation period, a statistically significant improvement in lower anterior face height (p < 0.01) was noted for the operated children. Thus, a normalization of the lower face height occurred throughout the total observation period. This would suggest that the neuromuscular changes which accompanied the abnormal mode of breathing were responsible for the initial large lower face height shown by the mouth-open group.

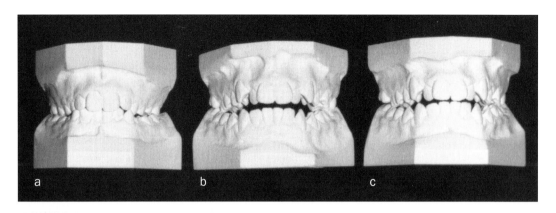

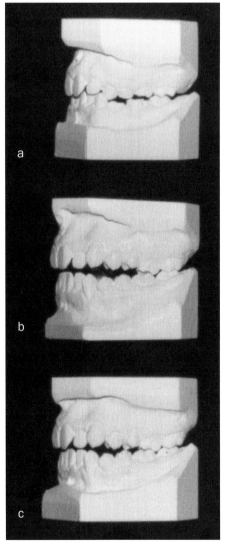

Fig 1-4 Occlusal deterioration followed by spontaneous and partial recovery from open bite after adenoidectomy in a girl between age 10 and 13 years. The initial models (a) taken in the mixed dentition show the case at 3 years preadenoidectomy when the incisor teeth were relatively straight and the bite closed. The middle set of models (b) shows the preoperative deterioration in dentition following 3 years of increasing nasal obstruction related to very large adenoids. The bite opened from the first permanent molars forward, and the incisor teeth were crowded. The last set of models (c) shows the improvement in the anterior open bite and crowding that occurred 2 months postadenoidectomy. Each set of models was photographed separately with the center of focus directed perpendicular to the occlusal plane. The three resulting photos were then mounted together to avoid any optical illusions.

Reversal of Symptoms Following Adenoidectomy and Changed Mode of Breathing

Figure 1-4 shows the dentition of a girl age 10 through 13 years. The patient had nasal obstruction problems in association with very large adenoids. During this period, an open-bite malocclusion developed. Two months after adenoidectomy and a change from mouth-open to mouth-closed breathing, the open bite decreased. This case illustrates how the mode of breathing may be associated with changed tongue and mandibular posture. It may represent one factor in the multifactorial complex that influences the dentition and morphogenetic facial pattern.

It is usually thought that the increased lower anterior face height associated with chronic mouth breathing is due to a downward and backward mandibular rotation. However, the same effect could also occur if the head is raised or extended in relation to the mandible. The distinction between these two concepts is important. Different muscles act when the head is tilted upward relative to a stable tongue, mandible, and neck complex compared with the situation that occurs when the tongue and mandible are lowered.[23] Thus, the soft tissue envelope of the face would be different in the two types of postural change, with possible differing effects on facial and dental morphology. For example, Solow and Sonnesen[85] have shown a clear pattern of association between incisor crowding and craniocervical posture. Subjects with incisor crowding in both arches had craniocervical angles that were on average 3 to 5 degrees larger than subjects without crowding.

A large number of studies have shown that an obstructed upper airway, in association with altered mandibular posture, is indeed related to increased lower anterior face height. However, some have questioned these conclusions.[97] One problem is that the correlations in many of these studies are small. A correlation of approximately $r = 0.3$ means that the association is of little value for generalized prediction. It is, however, strong enough to be noticed by experienced clinicians in extreme cases. These general characteristics of low to moderate biological correlations may well contribute to conflicting conclusions made in some investigations and review articles. In addition, those investigators who question the association frequently do not consider the three prerequisite conditions needed for malocclusion to occur in the presence of nasal obstruction. These conditions, as noted previously, are altered mandibular posture, altered tongue posture, and extended head posture. One or all of these conditions must be present for malocclusion to occur.

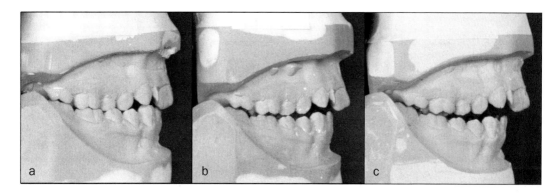

Fig 1-5 Change from Class I to Class II in a 14-year-old girl with excess lower face height. The centric relation occlusion is shown (a). The maxillary arch has been moved down 1.5 mm to imitate supraeruption of the dentition (b). This has caused a rotation of the jaw toward Class II. The maxillary arch has been moved down 2.5 mm (c). This has created a full cusp Class II and severe open bite. The illustration shows the large mesiodistal change in occlusion that can result from small increases in molar height in susceptible individuals. Obviously, these changes in occlusion can be reversed by small amounts of molar intrusion during orthodontic therapy.

Changed Mandibular Growth Direction After Changed Mode of Breathing

Orthodontists have traditionally studied dentoskeletal relationships in the anteroposterior direction and most diagnostic assessments are directed toward a horizontal evaluation of tooth and jaw relationships. Many malocclusions, however, are due to vertical changes in jaw position that can result in marked changes in anteroposterior relationships (Fig 1-5). If normal development of the anterior face height were better documented, the clinician would have a more effective means to evaluate malocclusions associated with increasing or diminishing lower anterior face height. Thus, population standards for vertical facial dimensions

have been prepared to assist the clinician in the diagnosis of vertical malocclusions. Such standards consist of:

1. Population standards for upper and lower anterior face height (Fig 1-6a) and total face height (Fig 1-6b) in a large population of Caucasian males and females established from ages 6 through 20 years.

2. These standards permit serial study of channelization for upper and lower anterior face height in a large population of both sexes, ages 6 through 20 years. Channelization means that the individual growth curve corresponds with percentile population standards (Fig 1-6c). If the individual growth curve crosses two percentile lines, the case is considered to be "not channelizing" (Fig 1-7).

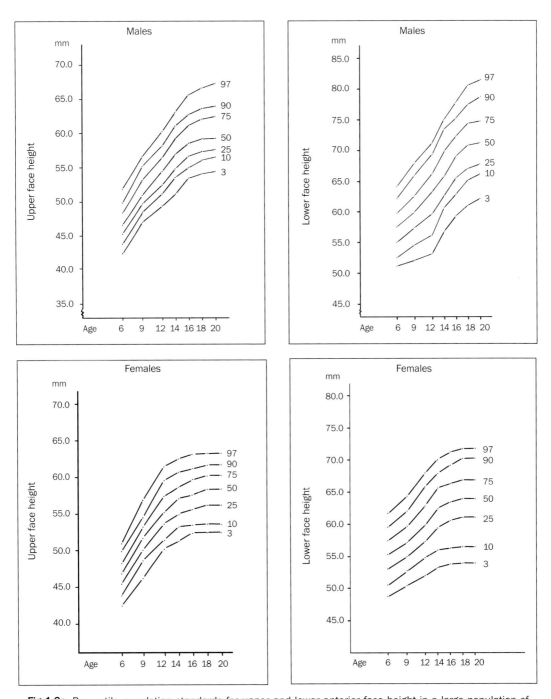

Fig 1-6a Percentile population standards for upper and lower anterior face height in a large population of Caucasion males and females from ages 6 through 20 years. The data are not corrected for enlargement and the enlargement factor is 9.84%. Upper face height was measured from nasion to subnasale. Subnasale is defined at the inferior point on the anterior nasal spine where the spine is 3.0 mm thick. Lower face height was measured from subnasale to menton.[102,103]

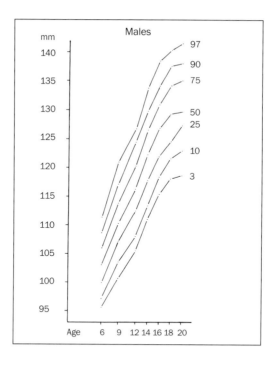

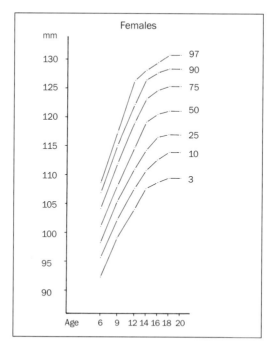

Fig 1-6b Percentile population standards for total face height in a large population of Caucasian males and females from ages 6 through 20 years. The face height was measured from nasion to menton.

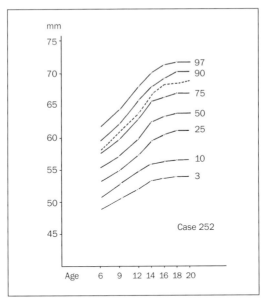

Fig 1-6c The dotted line shows that the serial development of lower anterior face height remained consistent throughout the growing years. Thus, the patient is said to channelize between the 75th and 90th percentile for lower face height. Such patients were found to have unobstructed nasopharyngeal airways.

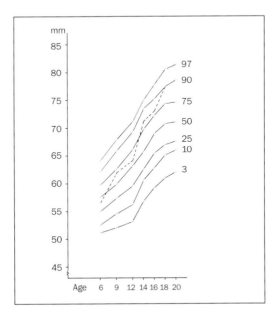

Fig 1-7 A serial distance curve for lower anterior face height relative to the percentile population standards. The individual patient, shown by the broken line, does not channelize and ascends from the 25th percentile. This patient had severe adenoid enlargement.

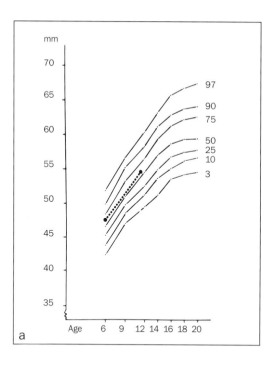

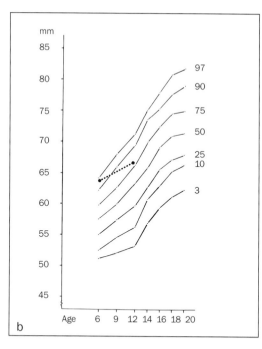

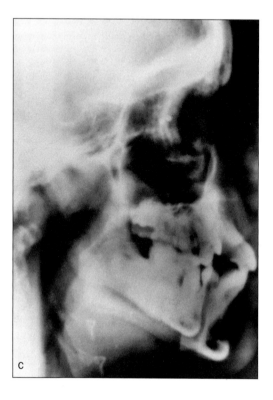

Fig 1-8 A 6-year-old boy before and 5 years after adenoidectomy who changed his mode of breathing from mouth to nose breathing. (a) The broken line shows the individual case plotted in relation to the percentile population standards for upper anterior face height. This shows normal channelization of growth in upper face height. (b) The broken line shows the individual case plotted on the percentile population standards for lower anterior face height. This shows a progressive normalization of lower face height from the 97th percentile to the 75th percentile during 5 years following adenoidectomy. (c) The initial cephalogram and the final one taken 5 years after adenoidectomy are superimposed on anterior cranial base structures. Note the horizontal mandibular growth direction and the increased labial inclination of the incisors in both arches.

Study of individual distance curves for lower anterior face height suggests that 18% of Caucasian males have either an abnormally large or steadily increasing lower anterior face height.[102] Such an increase could be considered a deterioration of face height relationships.

One case (Fig 1-8)[56] will illustrate how these charts are used to document the influence of a changed mode of breathing on the future development of lower anterior face height. The case shows a 6-year-old boy who had very large adenoid tissue and nasopharyngeal obstruction prior to therapy. After adenoidectomy, the mode of breathing changed from mouth-open to mouth-closed breathing. The upper face height followed the 50th percentile during the entire 5-year period following the adenoidectomy. In contrast, the lower face height was close to the 97th percentile initially, but normalized close to the 75th percentile during the 5 years after adenoidectomy and changed mode of breathing. One might speculate that improvement would continue beyond age 12 as the boy matures. The lateral skull radiographs also show a dramatically increased labial incisor inclination, thus providing space for tooth alignment. The superimposed cephalograms show the marked horizontal mandibular growth that accompanied this labial incisor movement. Without the change from mouth-open to mouth-closed breathing, it is probable that the lower face height would have followed its original percentile channel or worsened.

Furthermore, Lundstrom and Woodside[62] studied mandibular growth directions expressed at the chin for 260 participants in a Burlington Growth Centre study (serial experimental sample; see Chapter 2). They reported no horizontal mandibular growth vectors comparable to those found in the case described earlier. Figures 1-9 and 1-10 are from an investigation[58] where the changes in mandibular growth direction and the growth distance between the chin points were studied during a 5-year period following adenoidectomy and establishment of mouth-closed breathing. Measurements of mandibular growth direction and the distance between the serial gnathion points were obtained from superimposed serial cephalometric radiographs in 38 Swedish children ages 7 through 12 years with previous severe nasopharyngeal obstruction. These children were cleared of obstruction by adenoidectomy and changed to mouth-closed breathing during the 5 years postadenoidectomy. They were compared with the mandibular growth directions at the chin in a matched control sample of 37 Swedish children with unobstructed airways. The adenoidectomy sample initially showed significantly longer lower face heights, steeper mandibular plane angles, and more retrognathic mandibles than the matched controls. Analysis showed that during the 5 years after adenoidectomy,

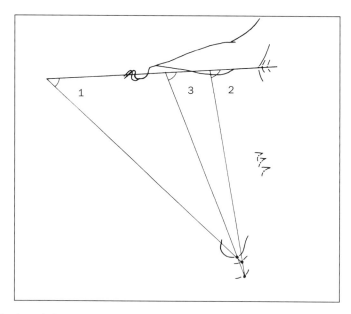

Fig 1-9 Determination of direction and amount of growth between structures from superimposed tracings made before adenoidectomy and 1 year and 5 years after adenoidectomy. The superimpositions of the tracings for each case were obtained by successive superimposition on the best fit of the contours of the anterior wall of the sella turcica, the dorsum sella, the planum sphenoidale, the cribriform plate, and the medial margins of the orbital plates on the frontal bones. The endocranial contours on each successive tracing were kept concentric so that a later endocranial contour never fell inside an earlier contour. A best fit for the sella nasion line was estimated for each complete set of tracings. This line and the individual subnasale and gnathion points were transferred to a single master tracing. The initial and 5-year postoperative subnasale and gnathion points were joined on the master tracing. This line was extended to intersect the common S-N plane and was used for subsequent measurements of mandibular growth direction, the distance between gnathion points, and the distance between subnasale points. The superimpositions of tracings are shown before and 5 years after adenoidectomy and, for the purpose of clarity, the intermediate tracings were not illustrated. Angle 1 represents the growth direction of gnathion during the first year postoperation; angle 2 represents the growth direction during the last 4 years postoperation; and angle 3 represents the growth direction during the total 5-year postoperative period.

the girls had a more horizontal mandibular growth direction than the female controls (p < 0.01). Although the adenoidectomy boys were statistically similar to the male controls, they also showed the same trend as the girls.

The growth separation between the chin points initially and 5 years later are shown in Fig 1-11. They were significantly larger for both the adenoidectomy boys and girls compared with the controls during the 5-year period after a changed mode of breathing. This finding can be explained by the relative mandibular autorotation and horizontal mandibular growth

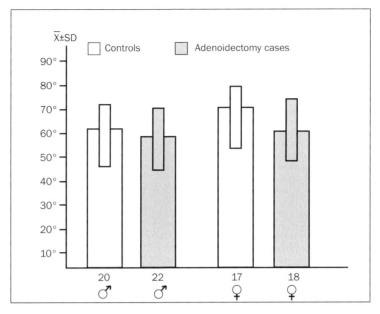

Fig 1-10 A comparison of the means and standard deviation for mandibular growth direction in control and adenoidectomy male and female patients studied during a 5-year period following adenoidectomy. The growth direction became more horizontal in both sexes and this change was statistically significant (p < 0.01) in females.

direction that occurs following a changed mode of breathing (Fig 1-12).

While much research has been directed toward mandibular changes, it appears that the maxilla is also sensitive to the adverse effects of these neuromuscular factors. Once again, the effect may vary depending on whether the child responds to nasopharyngeal obstruction by lowering the mandible, changing the tongue posture, or extending the head.[37, 58]

Dentition Changes Related to Altered Lip and Tongue Posture

It is thought that the dentition changes associated with an altered mode of breathing may take place under the influence of increased tension in the lips and cheeks,[81] plus alterations in tongue posture and mandibular posture. A change in tongue and hyoid bone posture in association with an obstructed nasopharynx and a subsequent change to mouth breathing has been noted in many investigations.[1,9,15,45,50,59,75,88,106] Thus, a change in the mode of breathing

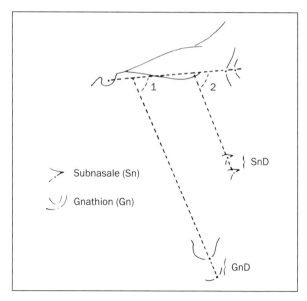

Fig 1-11 The initial and 5-year postoperative subnasale and gnathion points were joined on the master tracing, extended to intersect the common S-N plane, and used for subsequent measurements of mandibular and maxillary growth directions, gnathion distance, and subnasale distance. The superimposition of tracings was made before and 5 years after adenoidectomy. The mandibular growth direction is represented by angle 1; the maxillary growth direction is represented by angle 2. The distance (millimeters) between the initial and 5-year postadenoidectomy gnathion points is represented by GnD; the distance between the initial and postadenoidectomy subnasale points is represented by SnD.

may lead to a change in the balance between tongue and cheek pressures surrounding the dental arches. The altered tongue position may result in a reduction of the buccally directed pressure and if, at the same time, the pressure from the cheek musculature remains unchanged, the premolars and molars may be moved in a lingual direction. Fränkel and Fränkel[27] used this principal in reverse to explain how expansion of the maxillary arch occurs in conjunction with the use of his appliance. Thus, pressure from the cheeks is inhibited by the buccal shields of the Fränkel appliance so that the tongue can exert a greater expanding effect on the maxillary arch.

Incisor Crowding

Incisor crowding has traditionally been attributed to discrepancies in either tooth-jaw size or interarch tooth-size ratios. These concepts have led orthodontists to develop mixed and permanent dentition space analyses and in-

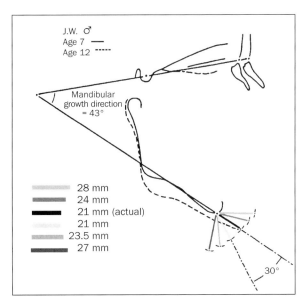

J.W. ♂
Age 7 ——
Age 12 -----

Mandibular
growth direction
= 43°

28 mm
24 mm
21 mm (actual)
21 mm
23.5 mm
27 mm

30°

Fig 1-12 Relationship between changed mandibular direction and the amount of mandibular growth expressed between chin positions during 5 years after adenoidectomy. The actual mandibular growth direction is very horizontal (43 degrees) compared with the means for Swedish male controls (62 degrees). The actual distance between chin points is 21 mm. The tracings show the effect on the size of this measurement with varying rotational positions of this patient's mandible. A severe vertical rotation increases this distance to 27 mm without any change in mandibular size. A horizontal rotation also increases the size of the distance between chin points to 28 mm. There is a critical range of approximately 30 degrees variation in chin position before this effect is seen. It is obvious that extreme changes in vertical or horizontal mandibular growth direction can produce an apparent amount of mandibular growth that has not actually occurred. Oral surgeons who perform Le Fort I maxillary impactions use this principle to obtain mesiodistal corrections in occlusions from Class II toward Class I.

terarch tooth-size analyses to assist in the diagnosis of crowded dentitions. Treatment plans have emphasized the removal of four premolar teeth in an attempt to stabilize the dentition. While individuals with large teeth may tend to have more incisor crowding, several factors other than tooth size may contribute to incisor crowding, for example, altered resting or functional activity in the facial and masticatory muscles.

In a previous study of the relationship between mandibular incisor crowding and nasal mucosal swelling,[105] cephalometric and dental cast variables from 30 male and 20 female children ages 8 through 13 years, with chronic nasal mucosal swelling, were compared with matched controls. These controls were orthodontically untreated and had no history of airway obstruction. The nasal mucosal swelling was confirmed with active posterior rhinomanometry and a head–out volume-displacement plethysmograph. The subjects with nasal mucosal swelling had significantly (p < 0.001) more mandibular incisor crowding than the controls. The normalization of incisor position after adenoidectomy[57] and changed mode of breathing were associated with a significant labial positioning of the incisor teeth in both jaws. In addition, Solow and Sonnesen[85] have shown a close pattern of associations between incisor crowding and craniocervical posture. Subjects with incisor crowding in both arches had craniocervical angles that were on average 3 to 5 degrees larger than subjects without crowding.

The change in incisor inclination that accompanies a return from mouth to nose breathing can be partly due to changes in tongue and orbicularis oris pressures associated with the transition from an open- to closed-mouth posture. Lowe[59] has shown that the anteroposterior position of the tongue is affected when the mandible is lowered. He found that the tongue progressively protrudes with increased mandibular lowering. Thus, an alteration may occur in the differential pressure exerted by the lips and tongue on the incisors. Lowe also found a highly significant correlation between the activity in the genioglossal muscle and overbite and suggested that the tongue's postural activity exerts a definite influence on incisor position. The complexity of these issues is further illustrated by the work of Takahashi et al,[91] which found that changes in body position from upright to supine significantly affected maximum tongue pressure during oral breathing. Their work also demonstrated that changes in hyoid bone position produced by changed mode of breathing and changed body position appeared to play a critical role in determining tongue pressure.

The following hypothesis (Fig 1-13) has been established for reversal of dental symptoms following adenoidectomy. After adenoidectomy, adenoid size is obviously diminished. This allows an increase in the nasal airflow and a change from mouth to nose breathing. This may, in turn, allow tongue position to be elevated and retracted. In addition, the head posture may change from an extended to a normal posture. The lips can then be closed. These changes in the neuromuscular environment of the dentition are accompanied by arch width increases. Furthermore, the labial inclination of the maxillary and mandibular incisors increases, the lower face height is reduced, and the depth of the bony nasopharynx increases.[53] Stepwise regression analyses support this hypothesis.[57,102]

A more labial incisor inclination and position after a change from mouth-open to the mouth-closed posture supports the concept of partial reversibility of malocclusion symptoms without orthodontic treatment. This change may provide additional space in the arches and thus assist the conservative alignment of incisor teeth without the need for premolar extrac-

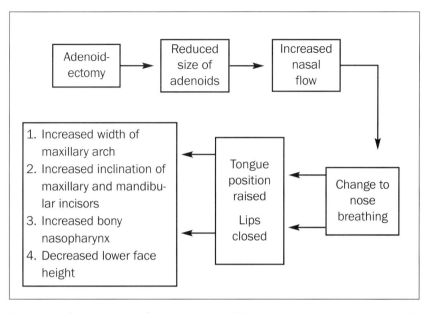

Fig 1-13 A hypothesis for the reversal of dental symptoms following adenoidectomy and change from mouth-open to mouth-closed breathing.

tion. Figure 1-14 shows a child with a changed mode of breathing. The models are at 1 year and 4 years postadenoidectomy. Note the space loss in the initial model. One would expect further space loss, since the deciduous molars have been extracted prematurely. Instead, spacing in both arches has occurred with increased labial incisor inclination. Some forms of incisor crowding previously attributed to tooth-jaw size discrepancy represent neuromuscular or environmental crowding, which may be partially reversible without treatment and may be treated without permanent tooth removal. The differential diagnosis of incisor crowding in young subjects requires an assessment of the degree of nasal obstruction secondary to nasal mucosal swelling or enlarged adenoid tissue.

Enlarged Tonsils and the Effect of Tonsillectomy

Behlfelt[9] has shown that children with enlarged tonsils as a distinct entity, unlike control children, also have more retroclined mandibular incisors, shorter mandibular arch length, narrower maxillary arch, high frequency

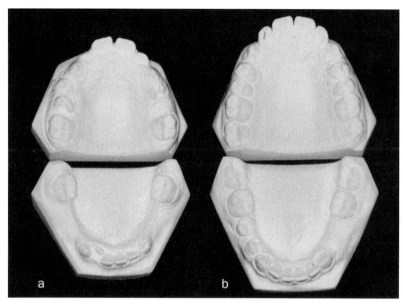

Fig 1-14 Occlusal views of maxilla and mandible from a male with severe nasopharyngeal obstruction. Model (a) was taken at age 7, 1 year after adenoidectomy, whereas model (b) was taken 4 years after model (a). The space available in the arches of model (b) is remarkable, particularly in view of the premature loss of deciduous teeth. It would be expected that space would be lost, but the reverse has occurred. This case is a typical response.

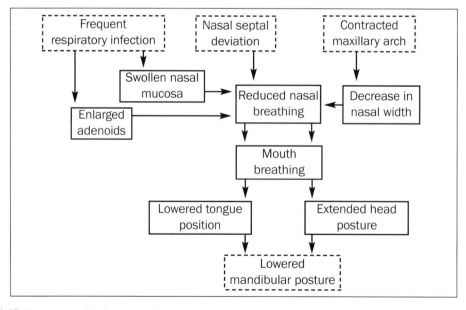

Fig 1-15 Factors contributing to the alteration in mandibular posture.

of posterior crossbite, large overjet, tendency to anterior open bite, more retrognathic mandible, larger mandibular plane angle, and larger lower anterior face height. These characteristics resemble those characteristics shown in children with large adenoids except for the large overjet. Enlarged tonsils that encroach on the oropharyngeal airway passage were shown to exert a strong influence on the sagittal tongue and vertical hyoid bone posture, and also on the mandibular rest position.

Thus, chronic alteration in muscle and soft tissue balance may affect the hard tissue morphology. Removal of obstructing tonsil tissue relieved the oropharyngeal airway passage. This allowed normalization of tongue and hyoid bone postures and also facilitated nasal respiration.

What Is the Mechanism Behind Changed Mandibular Posture?

The use of regression analyses has shown that a reduced nasal airflow or increased nasal resistance closely embraces related variables such as frequent respiratory infection, nasal septum deviation, and a narrow maxillary arch, all of which are associated with mouth breathing.[52] All these conditions may be associated with chronic mouth breathing, lowered tongue posture, extended head posture, and lowered mandibular posture (Fig 1-15).

Other Neuromuscular Adaptations Secondary to Upper Airway Obstruction

Changed Head Posture in Response to Altered Nasorespiratory Function

An important neuromuscular response that some individuals show in response to nasopharyngeal obstruction is an alteration in head posture. It has been shown by various workers that some chronic mouth breathers unconsciously maintain an extended or upwardly rotated head position. It is thought that this improves the oropharyngeal airway. In one study,[102] the head posture was investigated in 16 patients who had adenoidectomy because of obstructed nose breathing. A comparison was made with a similar number of controls of the same age who had normal nose breathing. In spite of the small number of cases examined, a significant difference ($p < 0.01$) in head extension was found when the two groups were compared before adenoidectomy. This difference was eliminated 1 month after adenoidectomy (Figs 1-16a and 1-16b).

Figure 1-17 shows that mouth breathers have extended head posture in association with excess lower anterior face height. Figure 1-18 shows the distribution of values for the upper

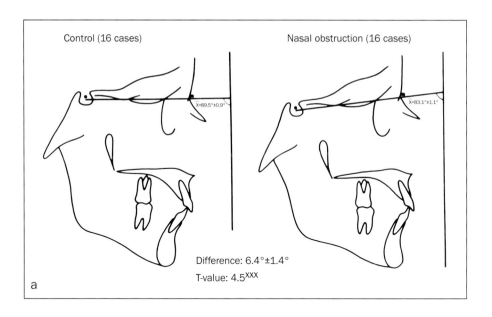

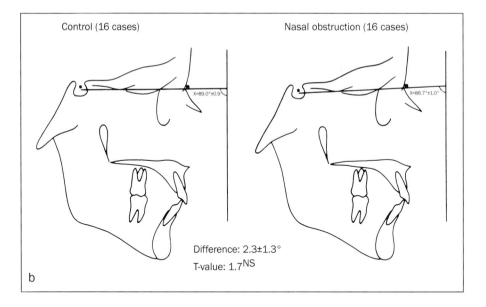

Fig 1-16 Head posture measured by sella nasion to a true vertical for 16 controls with clear nasopharyngeal passages and 16 children with nasal obstruction and mouth-open breathing before adenoidectomy. The head is extended in the obstructed sample (p < 0.001) (a). Head posture in the same patients 1 month after adenoidectomy in the previously obstructed group. The head extension has normalized and there is no statistically significant difference compared with the controls (b).

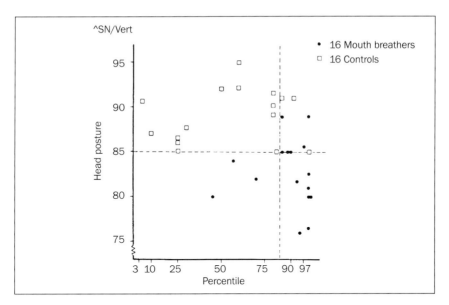

Fig 1-17 The relationships between head posture (as represented by the angle sella-nasion to a true vertical in degrees for Swedish children), the mode of breathing, and the percentile ranking for lower anterior face height assessed from Canadian population standards. The diagram shows that the mouth breathers are found in that part of the graph where the lower face height is large and the head is extended. The controls are found in the opposite part of the graph.

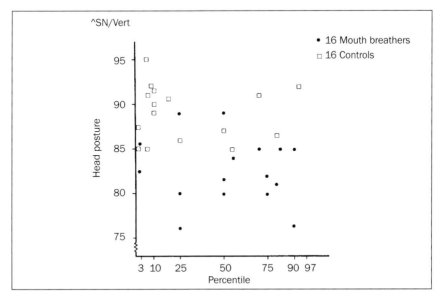

Fig 1-18 The relationships between the angle sella-nasion to a true vertical in degrees for Swedish children, the mode of breathing, and the percentile ranking for upper anterior face height assessed from Canadian population standards. The graph shows that the upper face height values for mouth breathers are spread over the whole range of percentiles. The upper anterior face height does not seem to be influenced by the mode of breathing and the head posture.

face height in the previous sample. There is no significant difference between the mouth breathers and controls in spite of the head extension and excess lower face height. This confirms that the primary effect occurs in the lower face. Solow and Greve[79] reported similar results and found head extension in association with a large nasal resistance. Vig et al[97] also showed that when nasal obstruction was artificially established, there was a gradual extension of the head posture with time. As soon as the mode of breathing was allowed to return to nose breathing, the head posture normalized within 15 minutes.

It can be concluded from these studies that head posture in patients with obstructed nose breathing is extended and this is associated with increased lower anterior face height.

Head Posture and Craniofacial Morphology

The physiologic changes already described can have a profound effect on facial structure. For example, Solow and Tallgren[86] found that individuals with large head extensions were characterized by large anterior face heights, and also both maxillary and mandibular retrognathism and steep inclination of the mandibular plane to the palatal and anterior cranial base planes.

In addition, a correlation study of predictive relationships[83] observed children for 2 to 4 years before the age of peak velocity in pubertal skeletal growth. They found that a large head extension was followed by vertical facial development. This was characterized by backward displacement of the temporomandibular joint, reduced growth in maxillary length, reduced facial prognathism, and less-than-average true forward rotation of the mandible. On the other hand, head flexion was followed by the opposite facial development.

Electromyography (EMG) has also been used to study this phenomenon. Hellsing et al[44] determined postural activity in the neck muscles in relation to extension and flexion of the head in adults. Both the supra- and infrahyoid muscles responded with increased EMG activity during extension and also with 20 degrees flexion of the head. Figure 1-19 shows this interrelationship between induced oral respiration, changed head posture, and the EMG activity of the suprahyoid muscles. Hellsing and L'Estrange[43] also used transducers to measure the changes in lip pressure on the incisors as individuals changed from mouth to nose breathing. They found that the upper lip pressure decreased when the patient changed from nose to mouth breathing, but increased during 5-degree extension (Fig 1-20). There was a clear correlation between lip pressure and cranial posture. Thus, in investigations of the effects of long-term alteration in head posture, compensatory

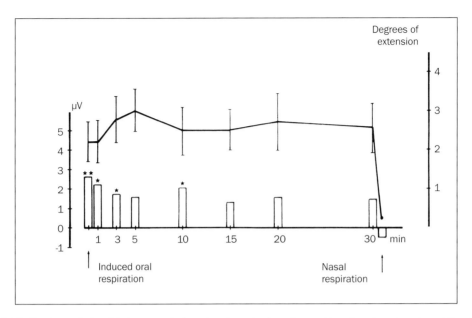

Fig 1-19 The interrelationship between induced oral respiration, changed head posture (———), and the electromyographic activity of the suprahyoid muscles (☐).[44] The graph shows that with induced oral respiration the head extended immediately and the electromyographic activity in the suprahyoid muscles increased. These changes remained until nasal respiration was restored after 30 minutes.

muscle function associated with head extension or flexion may be one of the determinants of craniofacial morphogenesis in growing individuals. These results support the soft tissue stretching hypothesis suggested by Solow and Kreiborg.[81] This stretching hypothesis is named after one of the links in the proposed chain of events (Fig 1-21). The coordination of different neck muscles is also important for adequate respiration and head posture. For example, if the head posture is changed by tilting the head backward from the lower cervical region, the nasopharynx will be narrowed. However, if the head is tilted backward from the upper cervical vertebrae, the nasopharynx will be widened (Fig 1-22).[42,84]

These findings indicate that airway obstruction triggers an increase in head extension via upper cervical vertebrae to compensate for nasopharyngeal obstruction. This facilitates oral breathing by enlargement of the naso- and oropharyngeal airway space. This head extension may create a stretching of the soft tissue envelope of the face and neck and thus initiate malocclusion.

On the other hand, such findings do not preclude that factors other than the stretching of the soft tissue facial

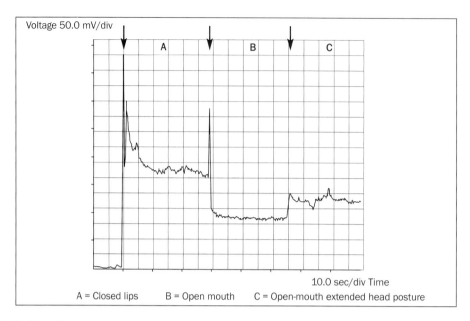

Fig 1-20 Upper lip pressure on the maxillary incisors measured by transducers. The pressure is elevated when the lips are closed. When the lips are opened, the lip pressure is reduced but then increases when the head is extended 5 degrees.[43]

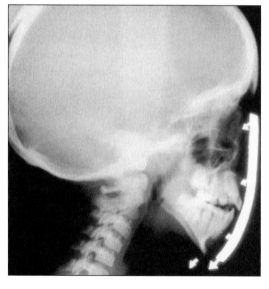

Fig 1-21 Soft tissue stretching and retrusive force on the facial complex due to an extended head posture.[81]

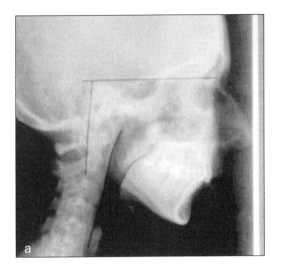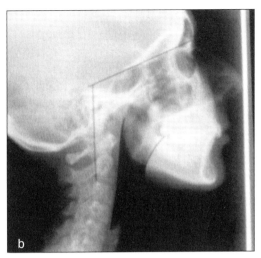

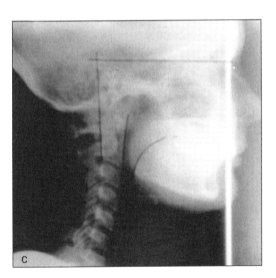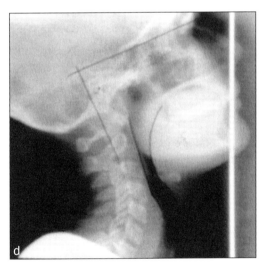

Fig 1-22 When the head is tipped up and backward the effect on the airway is different depending on whether the head is tipped from the upper or lower cervical vertebrae. Example (a) shows the width of the airway in normal head posture, whereas (b) shows the airway widening, which occurs when the head is tilted from the upper cervical vertebrae. In another individual, (c) shows the natural head posture. Example (d) shows that when the head is tilted from the lower cervical vertebrae the upper airway narrows. This distinction is important in individuals with obstructive sleep apnea so that the head can be arranged to open the airway while breathing. (Published courtesy of E. Hellsing.)

envelope could also be involved in transferring a change in head extension into an influence on facial development.[8,95] Thus, the head extension that accompanies upper airway obstruction also may lift the head and the maxillary arch away from the tongue. This, in turn, may have a narrowing effect on the maxilla.

The Relationship Between Airway Dimension and Head Posture in Obstructive Sleep Apnea Patients

Several studies have shown a relationship between the presence of obstructive sleep apnea (OSA) and increased lower anterior face height.[2,7,72] Solow et al[82] showed that the average craniocervical angulation in OSA patients was much larger than in six reference samples. They thus confirmed Hellsing's[42] previous findings. They also noted that when head posture is extended by tilting the head at the atlas the oropharyngeal airway is enlarged primarily at the base of the tongue and the epiglottic level.[84] On the other hand, when the head is extended from the lower cervical vertabrae region, the oropharyngeal airway will be narrowed. These findings may be important in the clinical management of OSA patients. Head support during sleep should be arranged so that the head is tilted backward from the upper cervical region. This principle can be combined with various intraoral devices to advance the mandible.[60]

Nonhuman Primate Experiments

Harvold et al[39] used nonhuman primate studies to confirm that a change in mandibular postural position influences maxillary arch width, vertical tooth eruption, and anterior face height. They showed that any factor which chronically lowers the mandible may cause an increased lower anterior face height. Induction of chronic mouth breathing induced in nonhuman primates was associated with maxillary arch narrowing, a decrease in maxillary arch length, incisor crossbite, increased lower face height, a steeper mandibular plane, and a larger gonial angle. These changes were most extreme in those animals that responded to the stimulus by lowering the mandible. It should be noted that some animals did not respond to the obstruction by lowering the mandible. These animals did not obtain malocclusion. When mandibular lowering occurred to facilitate oral respiration, it was followed by a downward displacement of the maxilla and increased tooth eruption. The key point is that changed mandibular and tongue posture are most important factors required for changed facial and dental morphology. Whether the air flows through the nose or the mouth is of secondary importance.

In summary, clear nasal airways are of great importance for jaw development, particularly during the early mixed dentition. Like nonhuman primates, humans may develop different ways to cope with nasal obstruction and thus the morphologic deviations may vary accordingly.

Controversies

While many studies document a clear relationship between airway obstruction and dentofacial development, some fail to demonstrate any such relationships. These contradictory results may, in fact, be in agreement. According to a current concept for the etiology of malocclusion,[80] the development of malocclusion can be seen as a disruption in compensatory mechanisms during growth, which adapts the dental and alveolar arches to variations in the sagittal, vertical, or transverse jaw relationships. When precise definitions of variables are used, such as a requirement that mouth breathing must be accompanied by a chronic change in mandibular, tongue, and/or head posture for skeletal and dental changes to occur, all well-documented studies indicate that obstruction of the upper airways leads to an increased vertical facial skeletal development. One would also expect an increase in the occurrence of anterior open bites under these conditions. This is not always observed because of the efficiency of the dentoalveolar compensatory mechanism that may adapt to the increased vertical skeletal dimensions by increased vertical development of the incisors and their supporting alveolar bone.

The reports of contradictory findings, made in surveys of studies on airway obstruction and dentofacial development,[96] simply reflect the absence of a theoretical framework for the detailed interpretation of the findings. The differences in opinion are also, in part, due to differences in sample selection and methodology as well as misinterpretation of data or results. For example, different methods have been used to assess the mode of breathing and nasopharyngeal capacity. These include visual examination, questionnaires, a wisp of down or cotton under the nose, vapor condensation on a mirror, roentgenographic study of the nasopharynx, rhinomanometry, anterior and/or posterior rhinoscopy, head-out plethysmography, nasal respiratory resistance, and simultaneous nasal and oral respirometric technique. Too much emphasis has been placed in some studies on different methods to assess the nasopharyngeal airflow or the nasal resistance. The individual's mandibular, tongue, and head posture response to nasal obstruction is far more important. Thus, alteration in mandibular posture in the presence or relief of nasal obstruction appears to be more important than whether the air flows through the nose or mouth.

Clinical Implications for an Assessment of Vertical Facial and Dental Relationships

Correlation studies[50,102] show clearly that the growth of the lower anterior face height is highly independent of growth in cranial base length, growth in mandibular length, growth in sagittal depth of the bony nasopharynx, and growth in maxillary length. It is therefore not possible to predict one variable from a knowledge of the other.

In addition, these correlation analyses showed that upper and lower anterior face height are independent variables. The lower anterior face height seems to be independent of the maxillary and mandibular skeletal units which comprise it[102] and, as Harvold[34] has shown, is dependant upon the mandibular neuromuscular suspension. The lower anterior face height is highly dependent upon mandibular growth direction[58] and those neuromuscular factors that influence mandibular posture, such as mouth breathing and head posture. It should be kept in mind that other possibilities, such as variation in the position of the glenoid fossa and areas not studied, may also have an influence on the lower anterior face height. Thus, considerable variation in the retrognathism or prognathism of the jaws is possible with minimal or no dimensional change in jaw size[5,104] (see Fig 1-12). These changes are possible whenever maxillary or mandibular position is altered in the vertical direction in response to environmental impact. The lower face triangle is used to illustrate this principle. It is formed by the maxillary and mandibular lengths and the lower face height (Fig 1-23).[35] There is a high degree of independent behavior between the growth of the components of the lower face triangle. In addition, a strong relationship has been found between the presence of airway obstruction and large or increasing lower anterior face height. These findings would lend support to the concept that some facial characteristics previously thought to be strictly skeletal or genetic in origin may also be created by environmental impact. This occurs when the highly variable lower face height increases its vertical dimension and sharply alters the anteroposterior relationships between the independently acting jaws, even in the presence of minimal growth.

The emphasis on the role of neuromuscular factors in the creation of excess face height does not imply that environmental impact is always a necessary prerequisite for excess lower anterior face height. This is because skeletal variables, such as positional relationships between the parts of the cranial base, may also be important in determining excess lower anterior face height. However, the strong effect of environmental impact on the neuro-

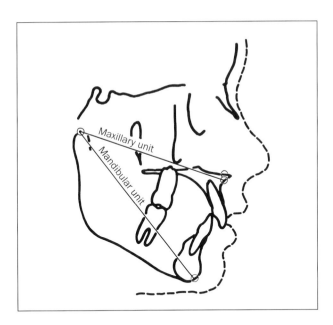

Fig 1-23 Harvold[34] has pointed out that there is a high degree of independent behavior between the maxillary and mandibular units. This is because the mandibular unit is highly sensitive to neuromuscular impact such as chronic airway obstruction, whereas the maxillary unit can narrow and its vertical alveolar height can increase. The unit itself does not appear to have the same vertical response to environmental impact as the mandible. Thus the mandible can rotate down and back to create mandibular retrognathism, long lower facial height, and an increased ANB angle when in fact the units match each other and no dysplasia exists.

muscular suspension of the mandible, and other dentofacial characteristics such as mandibular and maxillary retrognathism or prognathism, arch width, incisor crowding, and skeletal open bite associated with excess lower anterior face height, have been well documented.[5,50,52,105]

Changes in occlusion, incisor crowding/spacing, lower anterior face height, and mandibular and maxillary retrognathism or prognathism have also all been induced in primates through the application of a single, chronically acting, environmental impact.[5,35,39,64] In addition, similar changes have been shown in humans that were partially reversible after removal of the environmental impact.[52,58]

The ease with which such skeletal and occlusal changes can be initiated by chronic environmental impact and the complete or partial reversibility of the changes raises some interesting points relative to orthodontic diagnosis and treatment planning. The use of

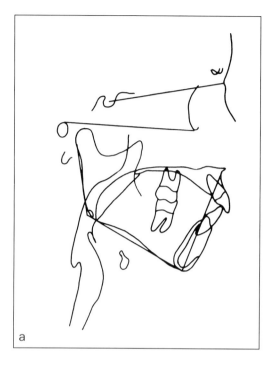

a

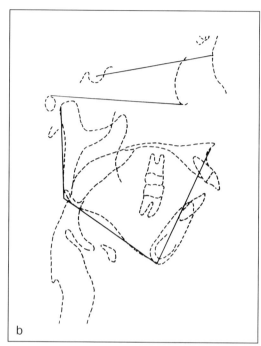

b

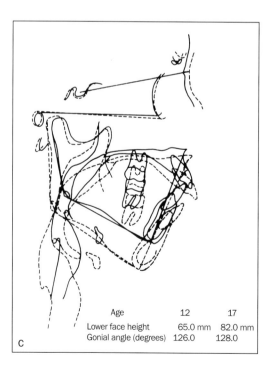

Age	12	17
Lower face height	65.0 mm	82.0 mm
Gonial angle (degrees)	126.0	128.0

c

Fig 1-24 The tracings show the dramatic changes in lower face height, mandibular retrognathism, and mandibular growth direction created between ages 12 and 17 by neuromuscular impact. At age 12 (a) the normal airflow through the nasopharynx was accidentally occluded following surgery. The resultant mouth breathing and downward and backward mandibular rotation at age 17 (b) was accompanied by the abnormal increase in lower face height, severe open bite, and supraeruption of incisor and molars. The superimposed tracings (c) show an abnormal mandibular growth direction that is down and back. There was an increased lower anterior face height from 65.0 to 82.0 mm. The tracings show clearly that some retrognathic or backward mandibular growth directions may arise from environment impact rather than genetic control. These changes occurred despite the fact that the jaws matched each other in size and no skeletal dysplasia existed. (Records courtesy of Dr R. Bushey.)

mixed dentition and permanent dentition analyses in the diagnosis and treatment planning of incisor crowding may be invalid procedures in cases that have environmental impact as the primary etiology. In such cases, narrow arch width, incisor inclinations, and incisor crowding may be partially corrected by a conservative treatment approach that autorotates the mandible toward more normal lower face height relationships rather than by an extraction approach. This concept is important in cases with excess lower face height and may also be important in short lower anterior face height cases with overclosure. Thus, in certain individual cases, a retrognathic mandible, vertical mandibular growth direction, open bite, and incisor crowding (Fig 1-24) may be primarily due to airway obstruction or other chronic environmental impact.[62] In addition such environmental alterations may also be superimposed on an existing skeletal dysplasia to produce very complex malocclusions. Such a concept requires a changed therapeutic approach from one that accepts the dysplasia and adapts the dentition to it to one that modifies the dysplasia by elimination or demonstration of the environmental impact and its resultant effects on jaw position, occlusion, and tooth alignment.

Three Data Samples

The data used to establish age- and sex-specific vertical dimension population standards for clinicians were derived from three samples:

1. The Burlington Growth Centre at the Department of Orthodontics, Faculty of Dentistry, University of Toronto, Canada
2. The Örebro Adenoid Study (Sweden)
3. The King's College School of Medicine and Dentistry Serial Growth Study, London, United Kingdom

The Burlington Growth Centre Sample

The 1,380 children who participated in this study were ages 3, 6, 8, 10, and 12 at the time the sample was initiated and comprised a cross-sectional control sample. They represented 85% to 90% of all Burlington children of these ages when the study was initiated. Three separate serial samples of chil-

dren from Burlington are included in this publication, which incorporates all children in the center for whom serial records were available.

The Serial Experimental Sample

The initial 3-year-old cross-sectional control sample became the serial experimental sample. They had orthodontic and anthropometric records taken annually from ages 3 through 18 and, in some instances, through age 20. These records included:

1. Medical examination and case history, including family and health history, nutrition, congenital defects, postural problems, and progress of puberty
2. Clinical examination to assess physical growth and occlusion
3. Facial photographs oriented in natural head posture

4. Cephalometric films, including lateral, posteroanterior, and right and left 45-degree oblique and lateral rest position films
5. Hand and wrist films
6. Impressions and wax bites for dental casts
7. Measurements of somatic growth: height, weight, length of trunk and limbs, breadth of shoulders and hips, girth of chest and abdomen, bone thickness, skinfold thickness, and handgrip strength
8. Behavioral data: a summary of interests, activities, opinions, and vocational interests

Some members of this sample received interceptive orthodontic treatment. Their measurements were always separated from the other groups until statistical analysis showed no significant differences. Naturally, the numbers for whom complete serial records were available diminished at successive age levels.

The Serial Control Sample

The children who were age 6 initially also had the serial records repeated at ages 9, 10, 14, and 16. The numbers for which complete serial records were available diminished at each successive age level due to normal attrition of the sample.

Cross-Sectional Serial Control Sample

The 12-year-old group from the initial Cross-Sectional Control Sample was examined again at 20 years of age and was known as the Cross-Sectional Serial Control sample. There were 64 males and 42 females for whom complete records were available. The Burlington Growth Centre sample was representative of the Canadian population in racial origin, family size, occupation, and climate. The sample was slightly higher in socioeconomic status and income than the Canadian average at the inception of the study.[14] Table 2-1 summarizes the total inventory of 1,380 children.

The Örebro, Sweden, Adenoid Study

This sample comprised 162 children from the county of Örebro in central Sweden. Of these children, 81 were patients and 81 served as controls.

The patients were all children born from 1955 to 1961 who attended the Otorhinolaryngologic Department of the Örebro Regional Hospital and were judged to be in serious need of adenoidectomy. Severe nasopharyngeal obstruction was confirmed by rhinomanometric measurements of airflow and nasal resistance. The distribution by sex and age for the adenoidectomy cases during this period is shown in Table 2-2. The majority of the

Table 2-1 Burlington Growth Centre Sample

(Ages 3 through 22 years; total inventory of 1,380 children)

Age	3	4	5	6	7	8	9	10	11	12
Males	132	167	161	154	149	144	141	141	136	127
Females	100	136	132	130	126	122	121	117	116	115

Age	13	14	15	16	17	18	19	20	21	22
Males	125	122	35	116	86	101	32	68	—	—
Females	113	109	0	103	47	86	31	57	1	—

Table 2-2 Distribution by Sex and Age for Adenoidectomy Patients (Örebro sample)

Age	5	6	7	8	9	10	11
Boys (numbers)	9	10	15	6	2	6	1
Girls (numbers)	2	5	14	2	2	5	2

children in need of adenoidectomy were approximately 7 years old. The sex ratio was 60% boys to 40% girls. During the period in question, a total of 166 patients underwent adenoidectomy at Örebro Regional Hospital. The 81 experimental patients were drawn from this group on the basis of availability of complete records.

The control group conformed to the age, sex, and number of the adenoidectomy children. Thus, the controls were selected by taking that child in Örebro whose national registration number came closest to that of one of the same sex adenoidectomy children. This means that the controls were similar in age to the patients. Further selection criteria for the controls were that they had no history of obstructed nose breathing, allergy, or recurrent otitis media and infections; they had never undergone adenoidectomy or received orthodontic treatment; and they were willing to take part in the study. The presence of a clear nasopharyngeal airway was confirmed by rhinomanometric measurements of airflow and nasal resistance. The controls were grouped according to the

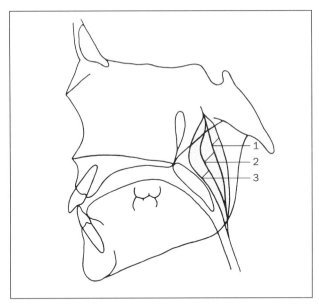

Fig 2-1 Size grouping of adenoids as studied on lateral cephalometric radiographs: 1 = no adenoids; 2 = small or moderate adenoids; 3 = large adenoids.

size of their adenoids as assessed on lateral radiographs (Fig 2-1) and consisted of 37 children with small adenoids and 33 with moderate adenoids. Eleven children with large adenoids were not included in the sample.

The adenoidectomy patients were grouped as 60 children with obstructed nose breathing and an additional 21 children who had adenoidectomy because of recurrent otitis media.

The King's College School of Medicine and Dentistry Serial Growth Sample

Data were derived from the records of subjects who had participated in the growth study at King's College School of Medicine and Dentistry,[11] London. Initially, 528 British subjects of Caucasian origin were examined at birth and 6 months.

Radiographic Technique, Enlargement, and Measurements

The Lateral Cephalogram

The Burlington Growth Centre

Six cephalometric radiograms taken with the high kV technique of Cartwright and Harvold[17] were available at each observation. They included:

1. Lateral film with the mandible in rest position
2. Lateral film with the mandible in the initial contact position
3. Lateral film with the mandible in open position
4. Right and left 45-degree oblique films of the mandible
5. Anteroposterior film

The anode-to-center-of-subject distance was 152.4 cm, whereas the subject-to-film distance was 15.0 cm for the lateral film. This gave an enlargement factor of 9.84%. The enlargement factor was slightly less for the 45-degree oblique films since the subject-to-film distance was 14.0 cm.

The Örebro, Sweden, Adenoid Study

The radiographs were taken with a Philips Rotapractix apparatus with a film-focus distance of 165 cm and a rotating anode tube with a focus of 1.2 mm. The exposures were made with 100 kV and 50 mA. The enlargement of the median plane with this arrangement was 6.5%.

The King's College School of Medicine and Dentistry Sample

The radiographs were taken on two machines. The first machine used during the initial years had a target-to-film distance of 183 cm while the second machine used a distance of 170 cm. There was therefore some variation in enlargement. The distribution of enlargement is concentrated very strongly about the central value of 7.76%, with 96% of radiographs falling within the range of 7.0% to 8.6%. All cases outside this range were rejected.

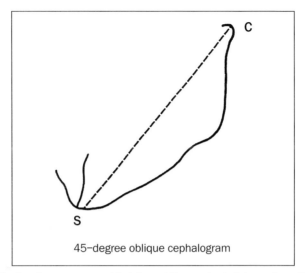

45–degree oblique cephalogram

Fig 3-1 The mandibular length measurement is taken at the greatest distance from the symphysis point (S) to the condylar head (C), measured to the nearest 0.5 mm. This measurement is used to represent the basal portion of the mandible and provides a more correct estimate of actual mandibular length than that obtained from lateral cephalometric radiographs. The head must not be tipped too far up or down from the Frankfurt plane during the radiograph procedure.

The symphysis point is defined as the midpoint of the inferior border of the mandibular symphysis. It is positioned in an area of minimal change in mandibular form and is suitable as a landmark to denote the anterior aspect of the mandible. Accuracy in location of this point on the 45-degree rotated cephalogram requires the use of the posteroanterior cephalogram to note the contour of the mandible at the symphysis point. The point can also be located by counting the roots of the canine and lateral and central incisor teeth. The symphysis point is then positioned midway below the roots of the central incisor teeth on the radiograph. The condylar head point is the most distal and superior point on the condylar head seen on the 45-degree rotated radiograph.

The 45-Degree Oblique Radiograph

Forty-five-degree oblique radiographs were used to make mandibular length measurements for the right and left sides of the mandible. These oblique radiographs were taken with an anode–subject distance of 152.4 cm. This radiographic projection was used since the head of the condyle may be seen unilaterally. It also provided a more accurate measurement of absolute linear dimension of the basal core of the mandible than was possible with the routine lateral cephalogram. This is due to the divergence of the rami of the mandible from the mid-sagittal plane. Although measurements of both the right and left sides of the mandible were made, only the right side was used for purposes of consistency in the preparation of population standards. The mandibular length was measured between the symphysis point and the condylar head (Fig 3-1). The symphysis point was defined as the midpoint of the inferior border of the

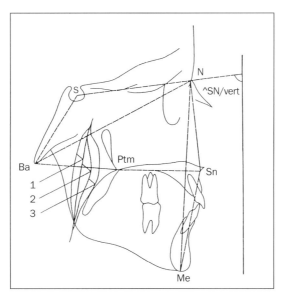

Fig 3-2 Grouping of size of adenoids: 1 = no adenoids; 2 = small or moderate adenoids; 3 = large adenoids.

mandibular symphysis. The condylar head was defined as the most distal and superior point on the condylar head. This method was sufficiently accurate for general clinical application. However, in case of severe mandibular asymmetry, corrected oblique films provide a more accurate mandibular length measurement.

Reference Points and Measurements for the Lateral Cephalogram

The reference points and measured distances are illustrated in Fig 3-2. The posterior cranial base length was represented by basion (Ba)-sella turcica (S). The anterior cranial base length was represented by sella turcica-nasion (N). The sagittal depth of the bony nasopharynx was represented by basion-pterygomaxillare (Ptm). The total cranial base length was represented by nasion-basion. The maxillary length was represented by pterygomaxillare-subnasale (Sn). The lower face height was represented by subnasale-menton (Me). The total face height was represented by nasion-menton. The upper face height was represented by nasion-subnasale. The head posture was represented by the angle sella-nasion line and a vertical plumb line in the cephalogram (SN/vert).

The sagittal depth of the bony nasopharynx was used to represent the sagittal size of the bony upper airway. The specific reference points and measurements are illustrated in Fig 3-3.

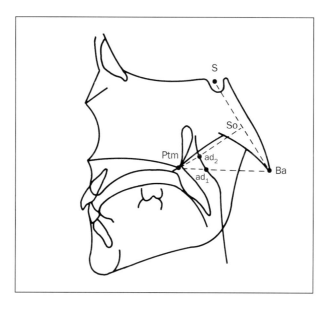

Fig 3-3 The reference points and distances within the facial skeleton used to measure airway size (Ptm-ad$_1$, Ptm-ad$_2$) and the bony nasopharynx size (Ptm-Ba).

The reference points are:

Ba = basion
Ptm = pterygomaxillare
S = sella turcica
So = midpoint of distance S-Ba
ad$_1$ = intersection of the line Ptm-Ba and the posterior nasopharyngeal wall
ad$_2$ = intersection of the line Ptm-So and the posterior nasopharyngeal wall

The following linear measurements of the upper airway were measured on tracings of lateral skull radiographs (Fig 3-3):

Ptm=ad$_1$ = sagittal depth of the airway through the nasopharynx
Ptm=ad$_2$ = sagittal depth of the airway through the nasopharynx at a higher level
ad$_1$-Ba = thickness of the soft tissue on the posterior nasopharyngeal wall along the line Ptm-Ba
ad$_2$-So = thickness of soft tissue on the posterior nasopharyngeal wall at a higher level along the line Ptm-So

Population Standards for Anterior Face Height, Maxillary Length, Mandibular Length, and Growth (Distance Curves)

It would be useful to quickly know whether an individual patient's mandible is large or small and symmetrical. Obviously, patients with large mandibles rotated down and back will obtain larger lower anterior face heights than patients with small rotated mandibles. In addition, it is useful to know when accelerations in mandibular size are likely to occur since these will affect the increase in lower face height.

Physical anthropologists have long been familiar with alternating sequences of rapid and slow rates of growth in relation to stature.[24,94] The linear growth of an individual or part of an individual may be shown graphically by plotting the absolute values of such linear measurements to obtain an S-shaped distance curve. When such distance curves are available for populations, they provide excellent methods for assessment of an individual's serial progress relative to his or her previous progress and to that of others.

Such distance standards indicate whether a child's size is within normal limits for his or her age, sex, ethnic, and socioeconomic groups. The channelization tendency of individuals to roughly follow a particular curve provides further information as to how far that individual has travelled along the path toward important maturation landmarks such as the prepubertal growth acceleration and adult size.

The smoothness of distance curves has led to the misconception that there is no prepubertal growth acceleration. A more complete picture of physical and facial growth is provided by plotting the same data as annual increments of linear dimension to provide velocity curves. Such velocity curves show that a prepubertal acceleration does indeed take place. When individual velocity curves are plotted, the growth acceleration occurs in a sharp fashion (Figs 4-1 and 4-2)[99] over a short period of time, in contrast to the mean curve, which is naturally smoothed by

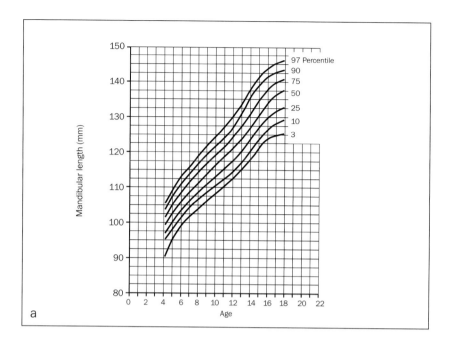

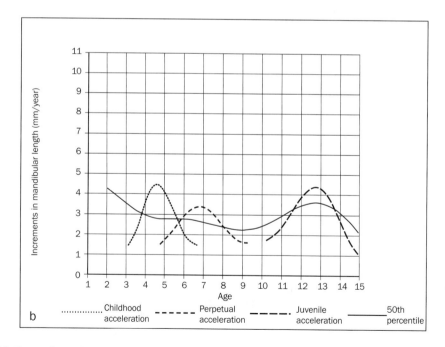

Fig 4-1 Percentile male population standards for mandibular length from 45-degree oblique radiographs (a: distance curves; b: velocity curves). Distance curves provide useful information regarding mandibular size and symmetry or good estimates of the amount of mandibular growth remaining.

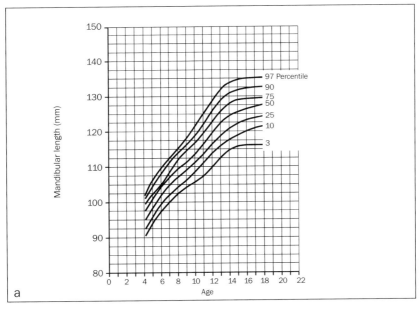

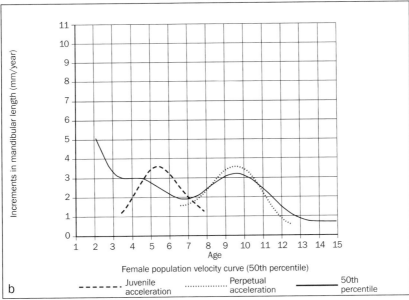

Fig 4-2 Percentile female population standards for mandibular length from 45-degree oblique radiographs (a: distance curves; b: velocity curves). Distance curves provide useful information regarding mandibular size and symmetry or good estimates of the amount of mandibular growth remaining.

Mandibular lengths that plot in the 90th to the 97th percentile area are invariably associated with Class III malocclusions due to mandibular prognathism. Such mandibular prognathisms may be camouflaged by mandibular rotation that may be associated with neuromuscular factors such as airway obstruction. When such factors occur, large increases in lower anterior face heights may result. Conversely, if a severe skeletal Class III malocclusion possesses a normal mandible, ie, plots at the 50th percentile, the case is probably a Class III due to midface retrognathism. Measurements of the right and left sides separately provide an estimate of mandibular asymmetry.

the averaging of a number of individual accelerations that occur at different chronologic ages. Tanner et al[92,93] have demonstrated this well, showing that some children mature or reach maximum velocity early while others reach maximum velocity at a later chronologic age. Such velocity curves provide a method to assess whether a child's rate of growth during the past year has been within normal limits for his or her age, sex, and ethnic and socioeconomic groups, and, in combination with distance curves, are useful in assessing the approach of the prepubertal acceleration. Since orthodontic treatment of dysplastic Class II cases should ideally be timed to occur with growth accelerations, once such accelerations are completed, the individual must be regarded as an orthodontic adult regardless of his or her chronologic age. This is because treatment must then be accomplished purely by tooth movements, rather than by the orthopedic control of rapidly altering jaw relationships during periods of active jaw growth. Accelerations in velocity may be noted qualitatively on distance curves as an increase in the slope of the individual's distance curve. These accelerations, however, are much less easily seen on a distance curve than on a velocity curve.

Tanner et al[93] noted that although children do not tend to stay in a given velocity channel during growth nearly so closely as in a given distance channel, marked change of velocity channel does signal an important acceleration or deceleration that is much less readily seen on distance curves. The velocity curve does require well-separated intervals between observations due to the large percentage error involved in small cephalometric measurements resulting from short observation intervals; hence, the distance curve may be a more practical tool for the clinician.

Nearly all researchers have attempted to predict a specific area of facial growth, such as the mandible, by correlating it with other craniofacial or physical characteristics. Tanner et al[93] have pointed out the necessity for serial observations on the structure to be studied. It would seem more reasonable, for example, to estimate mandibular growth characteristics using mandibular growth data, particularly when serial cephalometric radiographs are used. If the mandible is allowed to act as its own indicator of maturation status without reference to other craniofacial and physical characteristics, the introduction of unrelated variables is eliminated and the possibilities for individual prediction may become more attainable.

Clinical experience has indicated that favorable changes in occlusion and facial aesthetics are not as feasible in dysplastic adult malocclusions as when the individual is actively growing. In dysplastic adult malocclusions, complex mechanotherapy and orthognathic surgery must be applied to correct the occlusion rather than using growth in conjunction with a simpler orthopedic or orthodontic approach.

Once the visible signs of puberty are present, the maximum acceleration in growth is past, since puberty occurs on the downward slope of the velocity curve.[92,93] Obviously, it would be of great use to clinical orthodontics to be able to obtain a rough estimate of when the growth acceleration in various facial structures will commence.

Population Standards for Upper Anterior Face Height, Lower Anterior Face Height, and Total Anterior Face Height

Orthodontists have traditionally studied dentoskeletal relationships in the anteroposterior direction, and most diagnostic assessments are directed primarily toward a horizontal evaluation of the relationships of the teeth and jaws. Many malocclusions, however, are due to abnormal vertical development that can result in marked changes in anteroposterior relationships. If the normal development of anterior face height were better understood, the clinician would have a more effective means of evaluating malocclusions associated with increasing or diminishing lower anterior face height.

Normal population standards for upper, lower, and total anterior face height were established from large samples of both sexes from the serial samples of the Burlington Growth Centre (see Table 2-1). These population standards were assembled in a percentile format using the data available for the total sample. Thus percentile plottings were made at ages 6, 9, 12, 14, 16, 18, and 20. The variances of upper, lower, and total anterior face height were compared (Tables 4-1 to 4-6). Individual serial growth curves were plotted and compared with the percentile population curves so that the channelization of the upper and lower face height could be assessed for the total sample (Figs 4-3 to 4-8). The percentile curves show a steady increase in the upper and lower anterior face height up to age 18. Thereafter, a reduction in growth increments could be observed.

There were 22 males out of the total male sample whose serial distance curves for lower anterior face height followed the 90th or 97th population standard curve or ascended from a lower percentile to a higher percentile between ages 6 and 20. The development of these growth curves was analyzed in relation to the airway through the analyses of the nasopharynx and the nose, described previously (Fig 4-9; see also Fig 3-2). In cases with large (Fig 4-10) or increasing (Fig 4-11) percentiles of lower anterior face height, the following questions were asked:

1. Is airway obstruction in either the nasopharynx or nasal cavity associated with a large lower anterior face height relative to upper face height?

Table 4-1 Burlington Growth Centre Sample: Mean, SD, Range, and Percentiles for Upper Anterior Face Height for Males

Age	N	Mean	SD	Range	Percentiles						
					3rd	10th	25th	50th	75th	90th	97th
6	140	46.54	2.38	41.40–53.66	42.18	43.51	45.02	46.28	48.07	49.42	51.48
9	139	51.14	2.60	44.95–59.65	46.67	48.14	49.35	50.62	52.70	54.73	56.16
12	132	54.16	2.75	48.85–62.32	49.18	50.71	51.94	54.00	56.02	57.52	59.61
14	121	56.50	3.00	49.80–64.56	50.86	53.10	54.35	56.33	58.65	60.40	61.46
16	114	58.46	3.17	51.03–66.34	53.03	54.52	56.13	58.02	60.57	62.14	64.90
18	101	59.14	3.13	51.47–66.87	52.80	55.71	56.89	58.60	61.51	63.04	66.01
20	66	59.59	3.27	52.57–69.78	53.00	56.07	57.08	58.74	61.81	63.37	65.55

Enlargement factor: 9.84%

Table 4-2 Burlington Growth Centre Sample: Mean, SD, Range, and Percentiles for Upper Anterior Face Height for Females

Age	N	Mean	SD	Range	Percentiles						
					3rd	10th	25th	50th	75th	90th	97th
6	120	46.87	2.34	41.54–52.20	42.4	43.8	45.4	46.8	48.3	49.9	50.9
9	115	51.74	2.45	46.16–57.30	46.3	48.6	50.0	51.7	53.2	54.5	55.9
12	113	55.48	2.95	48.76–62.20	50.3	51.4	53.6	55.2	57.5	59.6	61.5
14	103	56.86	2.77	50.55–63.17	51.3	53.2	54.8	57.0	58.5	60.7	62.5
16	99	57.59	2.79	51.23–63.95	52.4	53.5	55.6	57.5	59.6	61.1	63.2
18	80	58.19	2.87	51.65–64.73	52.4	53.6	56.1	58.3	60.2	61.7	63.3
20	44	58.35	2.70	52.20–64.50	–	–	–	–	–	–	–

Enlargement factor: 9.84%

Table 4-3 Burlington Growth Centre Sample: Mean, SD, Range, and Percentiles for Lower Anterior Face Height for Males

Age	N	Mean	SD	Range	Percentiles						
					3rd	10th	25th	50th	75th	90th	97th
6	140	57.78	3.40	48.54–66.00	51.65	52.84	55.32	57.81	60.03	62.37	64.32
9	139	60.46	4.24	49.79–72.78	52.45	54.91	57.80	60.29	62.98	66.11	68.14
12	132	63.27	4.75	51.05–74.04	53.41	56.52	60.10	63.61	66.34	69.54	71.34
14	121	66.54	5.02	51.31–80.08	57.19	61.00	62.97	66.12	70.29	73.18	75.11
16	114	69.22	5.03	53.48–82.87	57.36	63.16	65.71	69.15	72.44	75.39	77.81
18	101	70.91	4.91	55.45–72.06	63.27	64.46	67.10	70.93	74.60	77.66	80.84
20	66	71.71	5.21	57.93–82.22	60.26	66.18	67.81	71.21	74.90	78.75	81.48

Enlargement factor: 9.84%

Table 4-4 Burlington Growth Centre Sample: Mean, SD, Range and Percentiles for Lower Anterior Face Height for Females

Age	N	Mean	SD	Range	3rd	10th	25th	50th	75th	90th	97th
					\multicolumn{7}{c}{Percentiles}						
6	120	55.08	3.36	47.42–62.74	48.7	50.5	53.1	55.4	57.5	59.4	61.7
9	115	57.51	3.58	49.35–65.67	50.5	52.6	54.9	57.3	59.7	62.1	64.4
12	113	60.19	4.24	50.53–69.85	52.0	54.8	57.4	60.0	63.0	65.9	68.1
14	103	62.46	4.63	51.91–73.01	53.3	56.1	59.4	62.4	65.7	68.0	70.2
16	99	63.23	4.69	52.54–73.92	53.8	56.3	60.6	63.5	66.4	69.4	71.3
18	80	63.91	4.88	52.79–75.03	53.9	56.5	61.1	64.0	67.0	70.3	71.8
20	44	64.62	4.69	53.93–75.31	—	—	—	—	—	—	—

Enlargement factor: 9.84 %

Table 4-5 Burlington Growth Centre Sample: Mean, SD, Range and Percentiles for Total Anterior Face Height for Males

Age	N	Mean	SD	Range	3rd	10th	25th	50th	75th	90th	97th
6	140	103.12	4.22	93.46–113.41	95.56	97.41	99.81	103.01	105.97	108.60	111.36
9	139	110.62	5.20	99.45–122.50	100.77	103.53	107.11	110.32	113.95	117.26	121.05
12	132	116.50	5.85	104.59–129.95	105.58	108.04	112.50	112.50	116.47	120.35	126.82
14	121	122.14	6.35	107.60–137.30	111.00	113.48	117.09	122.31	126.65	129.99	133.88
16	114	126.89	6.42	109.05–141.04	113.47	118.61	122.06	126.91	131.03	134.27	138.62
18	101	129.40	6.25	112.37–129.13	116.11	121.69	124.68	129.48	134.34	137.76	141.52
20	66	130.61	5.93	118.13–144.38	118.72	123.06	127.41	129.84	134.28	136.27	141.66

Enlargement factor: 9.84 %

Table 4-6 Burlington Growth Centre Sample: Mean, SD, Range, and Percentiles for Total Anterior Face Height for Females

Age	N	Mean	SD	Range	3rd	10th	25th	50th	75th	90th	97th
6	120	100.87	4.10	91.52–110.22	92.3	95.6	98.4	101.1	104.1	105.9	108.8
9	115	109.38	4.67	98.74–120.02	99.0	102.4	105.5	108.1	111.9	115.0	117.4
12	113	114.89	5.69	101.92–127.86	104.0	107.6	111.1	114.7	119.2	122.1	126.3
14	103	118.80	5.69	105.85–131.77	107.7	110.7	114.2	119.2	123.1	126.4	128.1
16	99	120.14	5.59	107.40–132.88	108.7	112.6	116.5	120.4	124.6	127.6	129.5
18	80	121.01	5.53	108.41–133.61	109.5	113.9	116.8	121.1	125.4	128.4	130.7
20	44	122.09	4.94	110.83–133.35	—	—	—	—	—	—	—

Enlargement factor: 9.84 %

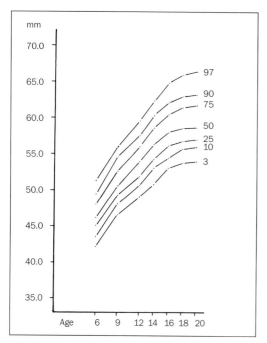

Fig 4-3 Percentile population standards for upper anterior face height for males ages 6 through 20 years.[102,103]

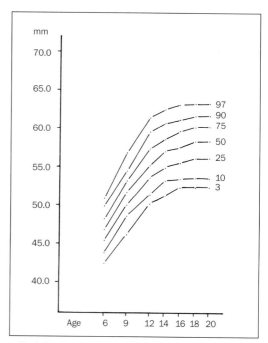

Fig 4-4 Percentile population standards for upper anterior face height for females ages 6 through 20 years.[102,103]

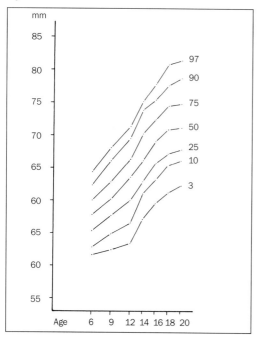

Fig 4-5 Percentile population standards for lower anterior face height for males ages 6 through 20 years.[102,103]

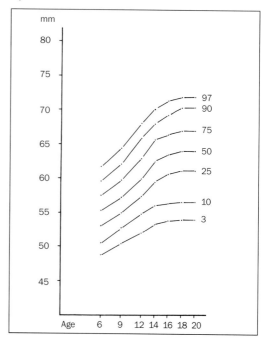

Fig 4-6 Percentile population standards for lower anterior face height for females ages 6 through 20 years.[102,103]

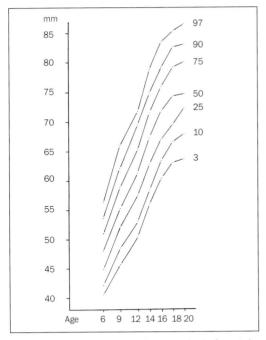

Fig 4-7 Percentile population standards for total anterior face height for males ages 6 through 20 years.[102,103]

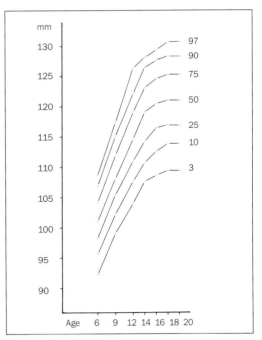

Fig 4-8 Percentile population standards for total anterior face height for females ages 6 through 20 years.[102,103]

2. Is airway obstruction in either the nasopharynx or the nasal cavity associated with an increasing lower anterior face height?
3. Is airway obstruction in either the nasopharynx or the nasal cavity associated with a decreasing overbite, ie, tendency to open bite?

The distribution of answers to the three questions for the 22 males with large or increasing percentiles for the lower anterior face height is shown in Table 4-7. From this table, it can be seen for question 1 that it is not possible to establish a relationship between a consistently large lower anterior face height relative to upper anterior face height and the presence of airway obstruction between ages 6 and 20. Neither can the airway obstruction be related to a decreasing overbite in individuals (question 3). However, the significant difference at the 5% level for question 2 shows a tendency suggesting that airway obstruction can explain why the distance curve for the lower anterior face height has progressively ascended from a lower to a higher percentile during ages 6 through 20 years in 16 out of 22 males.

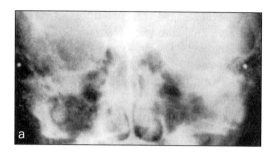

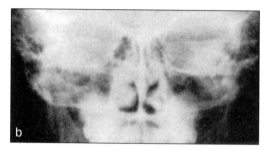

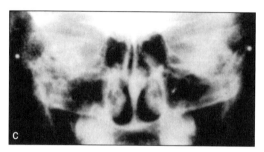

Fig 4-9 Severe nasal obstruction (a). Both sides must be radiopaque with no radiolucent areas throughout the majority of radiographs in the series. Moderate nasal obstruction (b). One or both sides show small radiolucent areas at various times in the radiographic series. Open nasal passage (c). Both sides show moderately large radiolucent areas.

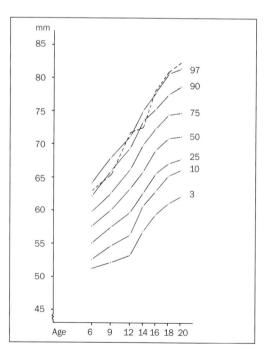

Fig 4-10 A serial distance curve for lower anterior face height relative to the percentile population standards. The individual curve does not channelize and ascends from the 90th percentile to above the 97th percentile.

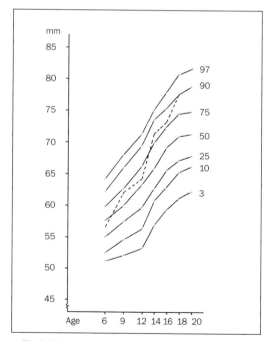

Fig 4-11 A serial distance curve for lower anterior face height relative to the percentile population standards. The individual curve does not channelize and ascends from the 25th percentile to the 90th percentile.

Table 4-7 Answers to the Three Questions for 22 Males with High or Increasing Percentiles for the Lower Anterior Face Height

Question	Answer: Yes		Answer: No		Difference for answers yes/no		
	Number	Percentage	Number	Percentage	Number	Percentage	X_2-value
1	13	59.1	9	40.9	22	18.2	0.72
2	16	72.7	6	27.3	22	45.4	4.54
3	14	63.6	8	36.4	22	27.2	1.46

The results shown in Table 4-7 may be influenced by the method used to study airway obstruction. Even if the nasopharynx and the nose seem to be obstructed on a cephalogram, it may be possible for the individual to breathe primarily through the nose. It was realized that temporary nasorespiratory infections and lateral rotations of the head in the cephalostat could give a false appearance of nasal obstruction. Correlation analyses show that the upper and lower anterior face height are more or less independent variables. The upper anterior face height seems to be primarily correlated to growth changes in the cranial base, whereas the dimension of the lower anterior face height seems to be independent of the skeletal units studied. This being the case, it is reasonable to assume that this dimension is highly dependent upon the growth direction of the mandible and those neuromuscular factors influencing mandibular posture, such as mouth breathing and head posture. It should be kept in mind that other possibilities such as variation in the position of the glenoid fossa and other areas may have an influence on the lower anterior face height. It could be hypothesized that considerable variation in the retrognathism or prognathism of the jaws[35] is possible with minimal or no dimensional change in the size of the jaws. These changes are possible whenever maxillary or mandibular position is altered in the vertical direction in response to environmental impact.

Changes in occlusion, incisor crowding/spacing, lower anterior face height, and the retrognathism or prognathism of the mandible and the midface have been produced in primates through the application of a single, chronically acting, environmental impact.[5,35,39,65] In addition, similar changes have been shown in humans that were partially reversible with removal of the environmental impact.[52,57,58,104]

The lower face triangle is formed by the maxillary length, the mandibular length, and the lower anterior face height. There is a high degree of independent behavior between the growth of the components of the lower face triangle. In addition, a strong relationship has been found between the presence of airway obstruction and large or increasing lower anterior face height. These findings would lend support to the concept that some facial characteristics previously thought to be strictly skeletal or genetic in origin may also be created by environmental impact. This statement does not imply that environmental impact is a necessary prerequisite for excess lower anterior face height. This is because skeletal variables, such as potential relationships between the parts of the cranial base, may be important in determining excess lower anterior face height, as well as susceptibility to alterations in the lower anterior face height subsequent to environmental impact. The effect of environmental impact on the neuromuscular suspension of the mandible and other dentofacial characteristics, such as retrognathism or prognathism of the mandible and midface, arch width, incisor crowding, and skeletal open bite associated with excess lower anterior face height, have been documented in other studies.[5,50,52] The ease with which these skeletal and occlusal changes can be initiated by chronic en-

vironmental impact to cause an opening of the mandible and the complete or partial reversibility of this change raises some interesting points relative to orthodontic diagnosis and treatment planning. The use of mixed dentition and permanent dentition analyses in the diagnosis and treatment planning of incisor crowding may be an invalid procedure in cases having environmental impact as the primary etiology. In such cases, the arch width, incisor inclinations, and incisor crowding that accompany mandibular rotation may be partially re-established by a conservative treatment approach rather than an extraction approach. This concept is important in patients with excess lower face height and may also be important in those with short lower anterior face height and overclosure. Thus, in certain individual patients, a retrognathic mandible, vertical mandibular growth direction, and open bite may be primarily due to airway obstruction or other chronic environmental impacts. In addition, such environmental alterations may be superimposed on an existing dysplasia or malocclusion. Such a concept requires a therapeutic approach that changes from one of accepting the dysplasia and adapting the dentition to it to one of modifying the dysplasia by eliminating or minimizing the environmental impact and its resultant effects on jaw position, occlusion, and tooth alignment.

Table 4-8 Burlington Growth Centre Sample: Mean, SD, Range, and Percentiles for Maxillary Length for Males

Age	N	Mean	SD	Range	Percentiles						
					3rd	10th	25th	50th	75th	90th	97th
6	140	46.45	2.25	40.76–53.47	42.25	43.89	44.83	46.44	48.08	49.33	50.12
9	139	48.38	2.81	42.26–57.13	43.56	44.81	46.39	48.12	50.37	52.09	53.73
12	132	50.67	3.28	42.98–58.30	44.83	46.60	48.49	50.86	52.65	54.66	56.26
14	121	52.27	3.72	40.04–60.94	45.58	47.37	49.62	52.28	54.67	57.25	58.57
16	114	53.46	3.63	45.26–62.12	45.86	48.42	50.76	53.23	56.24	58.15	59.15
18	101	54.71	3.85	46.36–62.86	46.51	49.13	52.24	55.10	57.57	59.27	60.69
20	66	55.60	4.16	46.54–63.38	46.97	49.49	52.90	56.06	58.36	60.41	63.15

Enlargement factor: 9.84 %

Population Standards for Maxillary Length for Ages 6 to 20

Population standards for maxillary length are presented in a percentile format for males ages 6 to 20. The data were derived from the serial samples of the Burlington Growth Centre (Table 4-8 and Figs 4-12 and 4-13). These figures show that the percentile distance curve for maxillary length increases up to age 18. Thereafter, a reduction in growth increments could be observed with the exception of the 90th and 97th percentiles. In none of the curves, however, could it be shown that growth was completely terminated by age 20, although this observation might be modified if data were available at age 19.

The distance curves for growth in length of the maxilla between ages 6 and 20 have different character and appearance to standard velocity curves for statural height for males. Growth in length of the maxilla would appear to occur over a longer period than is the case for growth in statural height in males. No appreciable pubertal growth acceleration of the maxilla occurs. The use of statural height developmental curves may provide insufficient information regarding the development of maxillary length.

A possible explanation for this finding is that growth in statural height occurs primarily as a result of epiphyseal growth in long bones and differs basically from the growth process pertaining to the maxilla, namely periosteal growth found in sutural and appositional growth. These two types of bone may develop under a different control mechanism and therefore respond in a

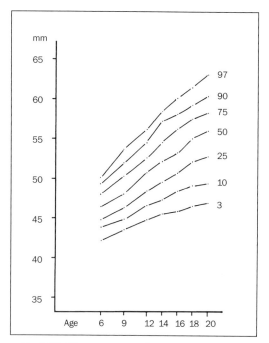

Fig 4-12 Distance curves for maxillary length for males ages 6 through 20 years.[54]

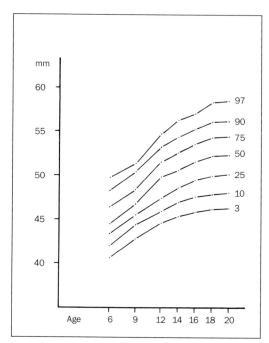

Fig 4-13 Distance curves for maxillary length for females ages 6 through 20 years.[54]

different way to hormonal changes occurring at puberty. It would be interesting to investigate in the future whether Class II cases diagnosed as midface prognathism show a greater amount of maxillary growth for longer periods of time than Class II cases due to mandibular retrognathism. In clinical orthodontics, the extended period of growth in maxillary length is important and should be given special consideration, particularly in cases of continued vertical development in the lower anterior face. It is particularly important in retention following

treatment of Class II malocclusions. Late maxillary growth may be a contributory factor in posttreatment changes in patients with vertically developing mandibles.

Population Standards for Mandibular Growth and Length

Modern orthodontic treatment planning can be improved with a knowledge of the following assessments:

1. Mandibular size attained at each biologic age (distance curve)
2. Knowledge of the channelization and variation in individual growth direction with age

Population standards derived from large serial samples of males and females from ages 3 through 20 can then provide reference material for the study of individual longitudinal growth to determine the true nature and predictability of individual growth rate.

Such population standards of the 3rd, 10th, 25th, 50th, 75th, 90th, and 97th percentiles by chronologic age are illustrated in Figs 4-1 and 4-2.[99]

Comparisons Among Standards for Vertical Dimension from Various Growth Centers and Races

Growth Centers

Since the data in the figures and tables in this text have been derived from different growth centers, the clinician will wish to know how these data compare with data from various growth centers and races. This chapter presents a comparison among data from the Burlington Growth Centre, the King's College sample, the Ann Arbor Growth Center sample, and studies of Asian and African-American populations. All of these data have been corrected for the different degrees of radiographic enlargement used at each center. The radiographic enlargement for each of the different samples is:

1. Burlington sample = 9.84%
2. The King's College sample = 7.76%
3. The African-American sample = 9.2%
4. The Japanese sample = 9.5%

Tables 5-1 to 5-5 and Figs 5-1 to 5-4 compare the values of four measurements for vertical facial dimension and

airway size. The Burlington, Ann Arbor, and Asian values have been corrected for enlargement, while the King's College values were already corrected. The Ann Arbor data were not included in the figures for clarity. The tables and figures show that the total face height measurements are quite similar between Caucasians (Burlington and King's College samples) and Japanese (see Fig 5-1). For example, the Burlington group is only 2.0 to 3.0 mm smaller than the King's College, Ann Arbor, and Japanese samples. The figure shows that African-Americans are a distinctly separate group with the total face height approximately 15.0 mm larger than the other groups.

There is also only a 1- to 2-mm difference between both the upper and lower face height measurements for all groups except African-Americans (see Figs 5-2 and 5-3; Japanese data not included). The latter have on average a 3-mm larger upper face height (see Fig 5-2) and a 12-mm larger lower face

Table 5-1 Comparison of Population Standards for North American Caucasian, European Caucasian, African-American, and Japanese Samples

		Total Face Height (N-Me)			
Age	Burlington	King's College	Ann Arbor	African-American	Modern Japanese
		Males (Means corrected for enlargement)			
6	92.97	96.6	93.1	112.0	–
9	99.74	102.7	101.2	120.2	102.3
12	105.04	108.3	107.7	123.7	108.3
14	110.12	113.6	113.8	129.3	114.6
16	114.40	118.2	119.4	134.8	118.0
18	116.67	120.2	–	–	–
20	117.76	120.2	–	–	–
23	–	–	–	–	123.2
		Females			
6	90.95	94.0	91.7	109.6	–
9	97.72	100.4	97.9	117.0	99.6
12	103.59	106.0	103.3	123.8	106.4
14	107.11	109.5	106.8	125.9	110.0
16	108.32	110.8	107.6	126.9	111.0
18	109.10	111.0	–	–	–
20	110.18	111.9	–	–	113.5

Table 5-2 Comparison of Population Standards for North American Caucasian, European Caucasian, African-American, and Japanese Samples

		Upper Face Height (N-Sn)			
Age	Burlington	King's College	Ann Arbor	African-American	Modern Japanese
		Males (Means corrected for enlargement)			
6	40.6	42.5	40.1	45.8	–
9	44.8	46.2	44.5	50.4	46.4
12	47.5	49.0	47.7	52.9	50.2
14	49.6	51.3	50.8	55.2	53.4
16	51.8	53.2	52.1	57.1	54.5
18	52.0	53.7	–	–	–
20	52.4	53.3	–	–	–
23	–	–	–	–	54.3
		Females			
6	40.9	41.3	39.9	46.1	–
9	45.3	45.1	44.0	50.7	45.0
12	48.7	48.0	47.4	53.8	48.3
14	49.9	49.5	48.3	54.4	49.8
16	50.6	49.5	48.6	54.5	50.4
18	51.5	50.0	–	–	–
20	51.3	50.3	–	–	50.0

Table 5-3 Comparison of Population Standards for North American Caucasian, European Caucasian, African-American, and Japanese Samples

		Lower Face Height (Sn-Me)			
Age	Burlington	King's College	Ann Arbor	African-American	Modern Japanese
		Males (Means corrected for enlargement)			
6	53.5	55.5	55.6	68.6	–
9	55.9	57.7	58.0	72.1	57.2
12	58.4	60.5	62.1	73.9	60.1
14	61.4	63.3	65.1	76.9	63.4
16	63.8	65.9	69.4	80.4	65.9
18	65.2	67.3	–	–	–
20	66.0	67.4	–	–	–
23	–	–	–	–	69.9
		Females			
6	51.0	54.1	53.8	65.7	–
9	53.2	56.5	55.9	69.3	57.2
12	55.6	59.0	58.1	72.4	60.5
14	57.7	60.9	60.3	73.5	62.6
16	58.4	61.8	60.5	74.2	62.4
18	59.0	61.8	–	–	–
20	59.6	62.5	–	–	65.3

Table 5-4 Comparison of Population Standards for North American Caucasian, European Caucasian, African-American, and Japanese Samples

		Upper face height (UFH): Lower face height (LFH) ratio		
Age	Burlington	King's College	African-American	Modern Japanese
		Males (Means corrected for enlargement)		
6	.76	.81	.67	–
9	.80	.84	.70	.81
12	.81	.85	.72	.83
14	.81	.84	.72	.84
16	.81	.83	.71	.81
18	.80	.83	–	–
20	.79	.82	–	–
23	–	–	–	.77
		Females		
6	.77	.81	.70	–
9	.81	.84	.73	.78
12	.83	.85	.74	.79
14	.83	.84	.74	.79
16	.82	.83	.73	.80
18	–	.83	–	–
20	.82	.83	–	.76

Table 5-5 Comparison of Population Standards for North American Caucasian, European Caucasian, and African-American Samples

Age	Burlington	King's College	Ann Arbor	African-American
**Sagittal Depth of the Bony Nasopharynx (Ptm-Ba)**
**Males (Means corrected for enlargement)**
6	38.9	39.8	41.2	37.7
9	40.5	41.2	42.3	40.1
12	41.6	42.5	43.6	41.3
14	43.1	43.9	44.7	43.4
16	44.2	45.1	45.6	44.4
18	45.3	45.2	—	—
20	45.2	45.4	—	—
**Females**
6	37.6	38.8	38.8	39.4
9	39.2	40.3	41.3	41.8
12	40.3	42.0	42.2	44.7
14	41.3	42.6	42.2	44.6
16	41.8	42.7	43.4	45.1
18	42.1	42.7	—	—
20	42.6	43.0	—	—

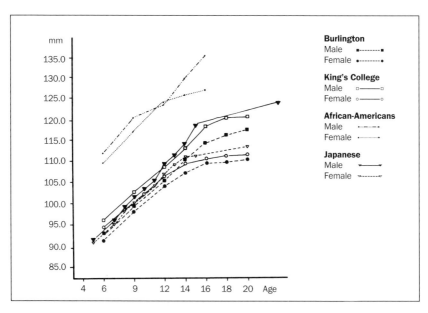

Fig 5-1 A comparison of population means for males and females ages 5 to 20 years old. The graphs show the means for North American Caucasian,[47,77] European Caucasian,[11] Japanese,[63,66,78] and African-American samples.[73] It is obvious that African-Americans comprise a different population compared with the other groups. Clinicians should consider the fact that the mean total face height for African-Americans is considerably larger than other groups. This is important when evaluation of vertical face height relationships is used as part of treatment planning. The data were corrected for enlargement.

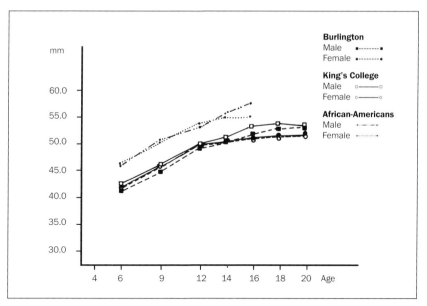

Fig 5-2 A comparison of population means for males and females ages 5 to 20 years old for upper anterior face height. The various groups are similar except for African-Americans, who have moderately larger upper face heights compared with the other groups. The data were corrected for enlargement.

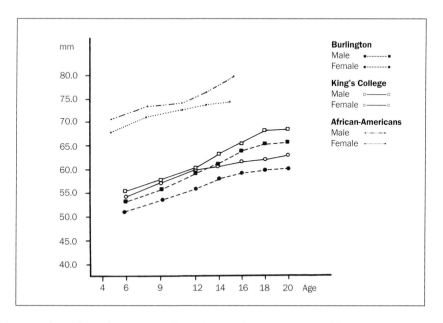

Fig 5-3 A comparison of population means for males and females ages 5 to 20 years old for lower anterior face height. African-Americans have markedly larger lower anterior face heights compared with the other groups. The data were corrected for enlargement.

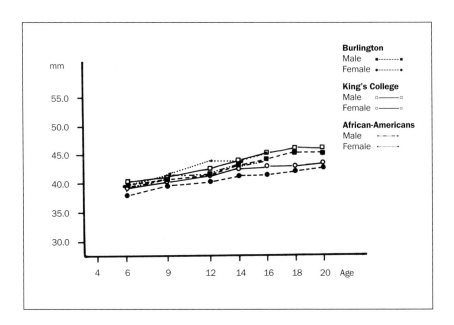

Fig 5-4 The population means for both sexes for the skeletal nasopharynx size are very similar among the various groups. There are, however, some sex differences for North American Caucasians and European Caucasians, with the males larger than the females. In African-Americans, the females are slightly larger.

height (see Fig 5-3). When corrections for the use of slightly different definitions for the anterior nasal spine (ANS) landmark are estimated, the difference between the values from the different growth centers is even smaller. This means that the standards for Caucasians are similar in different parts of the world and are quite adequate to use interchangeably for clinical purposes.

The ratio of upper face height to lower face height is similar for North American Caucasians, European Caucasians, and Japanese (see Table 5-4). The ratio for African-Americans indicates a longer lower face height in this racial group. Table 5-5 shows that the bony nasopharynx size (see Fig 5-4)

is similar in all groups. However, whether or not a difference in the size of the pharyngeal lymphoid tissues existed (see Fig 5-4) was unknown until recently. Recent work has shown that while Chinese have a similar bony nasopharynx to Caucasians, they have a larger pharyngeal airway because the pharyngeal lymphoid tissue is thinner.[109]

It would seem logical to evaluate dentofacial morphology for different races from cephalometric standards established for those races. This is thought to be correct because the various races originated from such differing geographic locations and climate conditions. This diagnostic problem is further complicated by the possibility that there are differing gene pools within the general classification of Asiatic or African people. For example, it is well known that Japanese and Koreans share many morphologic characteristics common to people of Mongolian descent. These characteristics may differ from those possessed by people of Chinese descent. Craniofacial standards for modern Japanese, established by Sakamoto et al[78] and Masaki,[63] have been shown to have backward divergent facial patterns, in combination with a small maxilla, compared with North American Caucasians. Recent work[66] has shown great dentofacial similarity between ancient and modern South American Indians of Mongolian descent.

It is important to understand the different dentofacial characteristics possessed by the different races today because people are migrating all over the world. These dentofacial differences among the races were understood during the early years of cephalometric radiography;[3,4,22,73] however, they have not received widespread use in North America and Europe.

Clinical Application of Vertical Dimension Cephalometric Standards

Figures 5-1 to 5-4 are derived from the data in Tables 5-1 to 5-4. These illustrate the differences among males and females in the African-American, North American Caucasian, and European Caucasian groups for some cephalometric measurements commonly used in the orthodontic analysis of vertical malocclusions. The differences among African-Americans and the other groups are noteworthy and confirm the finding of earlier studies.[3,4,22,73] It is obvious that separate vertical standards must be used for African-Americans.

While extreme variations in dentofacial structure can be found in any race, certain generalizations can be made:

1. African-Americans have larger dentofacial dimensions than other races. It is important to recognize this when linear measurements are used in orthodontic diagnosis.

2. The lower face height is proportionally larger than the upper face height in African-Americans compared with other groups. This is important when ratios of upper to lower face height are used in the diagnosis of vertical malocclusions.

3. The maxilla is more anteriorly placed than the mandible (related to the cranial base) in African-Americans compared with other racial groups. It is important to consider this when assessing the degree of dysplasia between the maxilla and mandible in orthodontic diagnosis. Thus, a larger dysplasia may be considered normal in African-Americans.

4. The angle of convexity is similar for African-Americans and Chinese, while the Japanese nearly approach the straightness of Caucasians.[4]

5. The Chinese generally have more retrognathic mandibles than other groups.

6. The dentition is more procumbent in African-Americans compared with the other groups. Chinese and Japanese have less procumbency than African-Americans, whereas Caucasians have the least procumbency.

7. The percentages of the various classifications of malocclusion differ in the various racial groups. For example, Class II Division 2 is uncommon in African-Americans, while Class III is common in people of Mongolian descent.

Nasal Resistance Standards for Children

If objective, accurate, and reproducible assessments of nasal respiratory function were available, it would facilitate the understanding and management of a variety of clinical problems approached by different specialists. For instance, the otolaryngologist would be aided in assessment and decision making when faced with the common question of possible adenoidal interference with the nasal airway and the appropriateness of surgery. Furthermore, the ability to monitor nasal therapy would add a much needed scientific quality to patient management. Similarly, allergists would be aided in the evaluation and the efficacy of their therapy. In orthodontics, many of the malocclusions previously considered to be genetic are now considered to be environmentally induced problems. This is a result of animal experimentation[39] and clinical investigation.[50] A steadily accumulating body of evidence[12,35,37,39,50] associates malocclusions characterized by excessive lower anterior face height with chronic mouth breathing. Active posterior rhinometry in adults[18,20] provides an objective dynamic assessment of nasorespiratory function that augments the findings of rhinoscopic, endoscopic, cytologic, and radiographic evaluation.

Diagnostic Rhinomanometry

Researchers first attempted to quantitate nasal patency over a century ago[108] because inspection alone was found to be inadequate for assessment of nasal patency. Rhinomanometry evolved as a procedure used to measure air pressure and airflow in the nasal airway during nose breathing.[48] This enabled patency to be expressed as resistance, which is the ratio between transnasal pressure and flow.

Active posterior rhinomanometry uses the head-out volume-displacement plethysmograph,[20] a technique

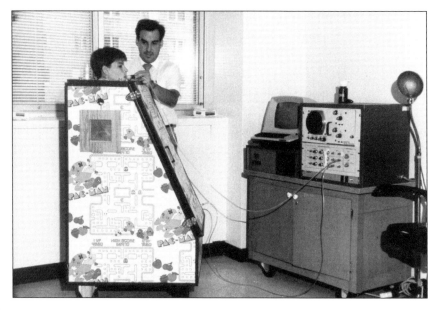

Fig 6-1 The head-out volume-displacement plethysmograph at the Airflow Laboratory, Hospital for Sick Children, Toronto, Canada.[68]

frequently used to measure nasal resistance (Fig 6-1). Active rhinomanometry, anterior or posterior, uses the subject's own breathing efforts as a source of pressure and flow. This is in contrast to passive rhinomanometry performed while the subject holds his or her breath and air is passed through the nose at a known flow to measure the pressure. Conversely, in this latter method, when pressure is known, flow can be measured. In posterior rhinomanometry, measurement of the pressure is made with a detector in the oropharynx as opposed to anterior rhinomanometry where the pressure detector is placed in the nostril opposite to the one being tested.

A volume displacement-type body plethysmograph detects changes in the volume of thoracic contents by measuring the amount of air displaced from the plethysmograph during thoracic volume change.[21,67] This volume change induces airflow through a laminar flow element in the wall of the plethysmograph. This flow bears a linear relationship with differential pressure that is measured across the element.[19] The advantage of the technique is that there is no distortion of the nasal vestibule with face masks, nozzles, or pressure transducers. Total unilateral resistance can also be measured when one nostril is occluded or when one nostril is completely blocked by anatomic deformity.

Respiratory airflow through the nose is predominantly nonlaminar or variable. Thus, its pattern of flow is termed transitional, a mixture of laminar and turbulent characteristics.[31] Disturbed flow promotes contact between air and mucous membrane ensuring warming, moistening, and cleansing. Changes in flow from laminar to turbulent result in changing mathematic relationships, which complicate the measurement of resistance. A review[21] of different instantaneous and time-averaged methods for calculating nasal resistances indicated a range in magnitude of about 25% among different common empiric methods. However, time averaged resistances showed less variation than instantaneous values.

Data were obtained from 1,000 consecutive patients referred to the Airflow Laboratory at the Hospital for Sick Children, Toronto by Parker.[68,69] These patients were referred by otolaryngologists, orthodontists, pediatricians, allergists, speech therapists, and maxillofacial, oral, and plastic surgeons who thought that there was a mouth-breathing problem. Dynamic assessments of nasal respiratory function were made to determine the presence, severity, and possible etiology of nasal obstruction and its association with mouth breathing. Respiratory airflow resistance was determined by active posterior rhinomanometry with the subject seated upright while a computer simultaneously monitored two parameters, transnasal pressure, and airflow. Transnasal pressure was measured via a peroral tube to the oropharynx, thus recording pressure between the oropharynx and the atmosphere during nose breathing. Transnasal airflow was measured by means of a head-out volume–displacement plethysmograph with a large laminar flow element in its wall. Five determinations of nasal resistance were made and repeated 8 minutes after topical application of a 0.1% xylomethazoline hydrochloride nasal decongestant spray. The highest and lowest readings were discarded and the remaining three measurements were averaged to yield the subject's nasal resistance.

The head-out body plethysmograph is much more acceptable to children than a face mask and the face and nasal vestibules are visible at all times. Alar muscle activity, including inspiratory alar collapse, is easily detected, while interference with facial tissues is eliminated.

After data assembly, the subjects were classified in one of five diagnostic groups on the basis of their clinical history, rhinoscopic examination, pre- and postdecongestant rhinomanometric assessment, and lateral cephalometric analysis. Subjects who satisfied criteria for more than one diagnostic group were allocated according to the major contribution to their elevated nasal resistance.

Table 6-1 Diagnostic Rhinomanometric Categories[68]

Diagnosis	Number of cases	% of total
Nasal mucosal swelling	317	32.1
Unobstructed nose*	295	29.9
Adenoidal hyperplasia	157	15.9
Septal deviation	93	9.4
Adenoidal hyperplasia and nasal mucosal swelling	93	9.4
Nasal valve incompetence	19	1.9
Postoperative pharyngoplasty	6	0.6
Undiagnosed posterior obstruction	6	0.6
N	986	100.0

*< 3.5 cm $H_2O/L/s$

The diagnostic classification was as follows:

1. The unobstructed nose: No obstructive pathology was evident on rhinoscopic examination and the predecongestant values approached those of the healthy adult. An upper limit for normal nasal resistance of 3.5 cm $H_2O/L/s$ was assigned.
2. Nasal mucosal swelling: Nasal resistance of the predecongestant nose was markedly elevated, varying between 5 and 15 cm $H_2O/L/s$, and was substantially reduced by decongestant spray.
3. Nasal skeletal abnormality: To determine the effect of bony and/or cartilaginous septal deviation on nasal airflow, the nasal cavities were tested individually and together after a decongestant spray and the two sides were compared.
4. Adenoidal obstruction: A standardized lateral head film was taken to confirm the presence of adenoid tissue in relation to the size of the bony nasopharynx. When adenoid tissue occluded the nasopharyngeal airway, the nasal resistance was not reduced by nasal decongestant spray. If the initial rhinoscopic examination excluded other causes of obstruction, for example, septal deviation, the diagnosis of adenoidal obstruction was accepted.
5. Nasal valve incompetence: Elevated nasal resistance was reduced substantially after wide retraction of the nasal alar. In a healthy adult nose, alar retraction halved nasal resistance.

Table 6-1 is very important because it shows the percentages of the different diagnostic categories in a large population of Canadian children. The most frequent diagnosis was nasal mucosal swelling, which composed 32.1% of the sample. Adenoid hypertrophy was approximately one half as

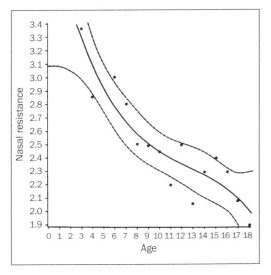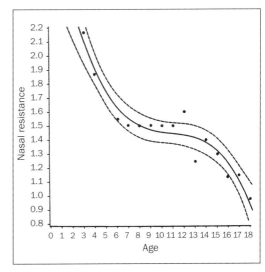

Fig 6-2 Nasal resistance as a function of age plus the 95% confidence limits for a sample of individuals with unobstructed nasopharyngeal airways from ages 3 through 18.[69]

frequent (15.9%). A surprising finding was that 29.9% of patients who were referred because of mouth breathing and suspected elevated nasal resistance had normal values equal to or less than 3.5 cm $H_2O/L/s$. In these children, the etiology of the mouth-open posture was probably habit.

One of the most important points for the clinician to understand is illustrated in Fig 6-2. These linear regression analyses show that with every year of increased age, one can expect an annual average improvement in nasal resistance in children of both sexes. This improvement is explained in Fig 6-3, which shows that the nasopharyngeal lymphoid tissue decreases with age, while the size of the nasopharyngeal airway increases with age.[55]

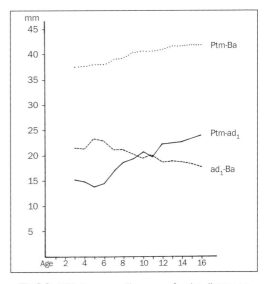

Fig 6-3 Fiftieth percentile curves for the distances Ptm-Ba, Ptm-ad$_1$, and ad$_1$-Ba in boys and girls. The table shows that the nasopharyngeal lymphoid tissue (ad$_1$-Ba) decreases in size with age, whereas the bony nasopharynx and the nasopharyngeal airway (Ptm-ad$_1$, Ptm-Ba) increase.

Clinical Application of Vertical Change in the Jaws and Dentition

chapter

7

Figures 7-1[62,102] and 1-24 and Table 7-1 illustrate an important point in orthodontic treatment planning: Many mesiodistal changes in the dentition and jaw relationships are achieved by a vertical manipulation of the dentition. This concept implies that orthodontic treatment is able to modify the original skeletal pattern presented by some patients.

In contrast to this concept, most conventional orthodontic thought has assumed that the skeletal pattern of individual patients is immutable and not susceptible to change by therapy. Thus, orthodontic treatment is frequently directed to an adaptation of the dentition to the existing skeletal pattern or its predicted future growth. These adaptations are obtained through the use of extractions, headgear therapy, and Class II elastics. Few treatment plans aim to modify an existing mandibular growth direction to a more favorable one prior to or during orthodontic therapy by means of applied biology.

Our work shows clearly that changed mode of breathing is one factor that may contribute to change from vertical to horizontal mandibular growth direction (Fig 7-2).[58] This will have a profound effect on mandibular retrognathism or prognathism as is shown in Fig 1-12,[104] which illustrates that varying rotational positions of identical-length mandibles produce different distances between the chin points on superimposed tracings. The illustration shows that changes from a vertical to a horizontal mandibular growth posture (or the reverse) can produce an increased distance between chin positions, which is unrelated to any increased mandibular length. Le Fort I surgical impaction of the maxilla also illustrates this principle when vertical changes in maxillary alveolar height allow mandibular autorotation from Class II toward Class I. Thus, in Class II cases when the mandible is rotated up and forward following surgical impaction of the max-

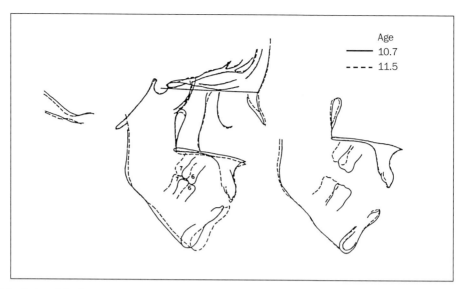

Fig 7-1 Patient C.L. illustrates an anterior open bite that has been partially corrected by an orthodontically created upward and forward mandibular rotation. This rotation was created by inhibition of buccal segment eruption following the establishment of nose breathing. The appliance used was a posterior occlusal bite block that prevented molar eruption while the breathing and jaw position normalized. The resultant mandibular growth direction was 16 degrees anteriorly when measured to SN. When one considers that the mean for a large sample of Canadian females was 74 degrees and the most horizontally growing mandible in the entire female sample was 47 degrees, the changes seen in this patient can be attributed only to therapy. Thus, change in mandibular prognathism can be achieved even with a minimal change in jaw size.[62] (Teeth numbered according to Palmer Notation System.)

Table 7-1 Patient C.L.

Age	SNA	SNB	ANB (degrees)	I to NB (degrees)	Pg to NB (degrees)	LFH	Md-Mx Diff
10.7	77.0	72.0	5.0	6.5	2.5	69.5	23.0
11.5	76.5	74.5	2.0	6.5	2.5	67.5	24.0

(Measurements in mm, unless noted otherwise)

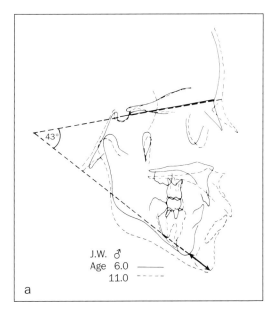

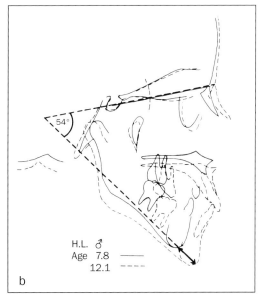

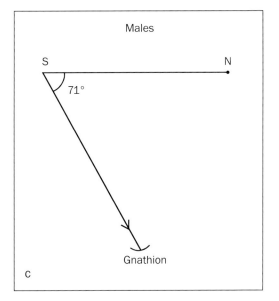

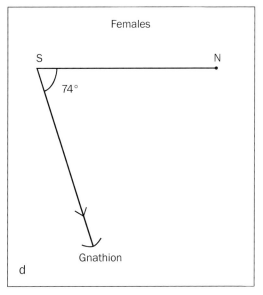

Fig 7-2 Large amounts of horizontal mandibular growth expressed at the chin 5 years after adenoidectomy on two boys who changed from mouth-open to mouth-closed breathing after adenoidectomy (a, b). When these growth directions are compared with the mean mandibular growth directions for a sample of 117 Canadian males and 109 Canadian females (c, d), the effect on the mandibular growth direction is obvious. No orthodontic treatment was performed.[104]

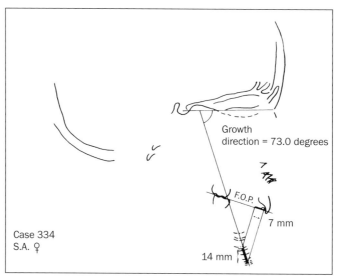

Growth
direction = 73.0 degrees

F.O.P.

7 mm

Case 334
S.A. ♀

14 mm

Fig 7-3 Mandibular growth direction found in an untreated child from the Burlington Growth Centre sample where the growth direction is the same as the means for mandibular growth direction for the Burlington Growth Centre. The figure, with superimpositions annually from age 6 to 16, shows that in the absence of any forward maxillary growth or tooth movement, 14.0 mm of mandibular growth expressed at the chin over 5.5 years could be required to give a 7.0-mm correction along the occlusal plane. With a more horizontal mandibular growth direction, less growth would be required to produce 7.0 mm of change on the occlusal plane. If forward maxillary growth occurred, even more mandibular growth would be required. This figure illustrates the point that with the usual mandibular growth direction found in the population, large amounts of mandibular growth are required to produce small mesiodistal corrections within the dentition. If a horizontal mandibular growth direction is combined with the effect of extra growth expressed at the chin, fewer millimeters of mandibular growth in length will be required to provide a 7.0-mm Class II correction along the functional occlusal plane.[104]

illa, the occlusion changes from Class II toward Class I purely as a result of this rotational phenomenon. In vertically rotating mandibles, this effect becomes increasingly deleterious to the face. It is, however, beneficial when horizontal growth directions are produced. Thus, small changes in molar height will be accompanied by large changes in mesiodistal occlusion, as seen in Fig 1-5, where small increases in maxillary molar height have changed the case from Class I to complete Class II.

Few cephalometric analyses and growth prediction systems recognize this phenomena. An understanding of the factors that can increase or decrease the lower anterior face height will enable the clinician to correctly plan orthodontic treatment from a few selected measurements of vertical facial dimensions.

Our previous studies[58] have shown that children with previous severe nasopharyngeal obstruction may have more horizontally growing mandibles after the change from mouth-open to mouth-closed breathing. When one combines this change with a more horizontally positioned mandible, the clin-

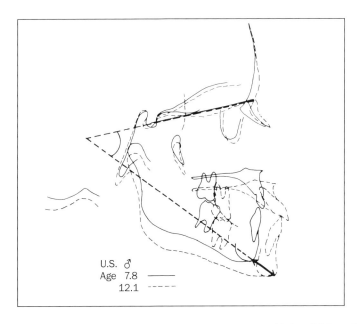

Fig 7-4 Note the progressive improvement in face-height proportionality (13.2 to 28.0 mm). The upper face height continued to increase while the lower did not, noteworthy behavior in an area that is supposed to change greatly during 5 years of growth.

ical implications are interesting. For example, there has been a great deal of debate about the possibility of increasing mandibular length with functional appliances. Even if these length increases can be ensured, they may have a small or negligible effect in correcting a Class II malocclusion. This is because the malocclusion is usually corrected mesiodistally along the functional occlusal plane, which is not parallel to the usual mandibular growth direction. As Fig 7-3 shows, specific patients may need many millimeters of downward and forward mandibular growth to achieve a 7-mm mesiodistal correction along the occlusal plane where mesiodistal occlusal corrections occur. If forward maxillary

growth occurs, even more millimeters of mandibular growth will be required to achieve the correction. Rather than attempting to obtain a few millimeters of increased mandibular length, a better approach to the orthodontic treatment of Class II malocclusions characterized by excess lower face height is to imitate increased mandibular growth by directing that growth in a more horizontal direction after correcting the etiologic biology.

Figure 7-4 and Table 7-2 illustrate the application of this approach. The boy in Fig 7-4 shows dramatic improvement in the ratio of upper face height to lower face height where the ratio changed from .76 to .94. This improvement took place over 5 years, following

Table 7-2 Growth Directed More Horizontally to Imitate Mandibular Growth: Patient US Male

Age	UFH:LFH ratio	Airway size	Bony pharyngeal size	UFH	LFH
7	.76	13.2	43.4	43.0	54.0
8	.84	—	—	45.5	54.0
12	.94	28.0	44.3	52.5	56.0

(Measurements in mm)

Table 7-3 Patient D.R. (male; 16 years, 8 months)

	ANB (degrees)	Md U	Mx U	Diff	LFH	UFH:LFH ratio
Standard	2.0	127	100	27	71	.80
Patient	3.5	126	96	30	88	.69

(Measurements in mm, unless noted otherwise)

Table 7-4 Patient D.R.

Age	ANB (degrees)	Md U	Mx U	Diff	LFH	UFH:LFH ratio
16.8	3.5	126	96	34	88	.69
19.0	1.0	134	100	34	84	.73

(Measurements in mm, unless noted otherwise)

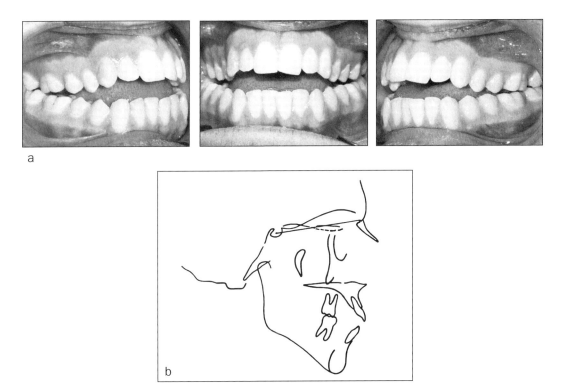

Figs 7-5a and 7-5b The illustrations show the before-treatment records of patient D.R. age 16 years and 8 months with a retrognathic mandible, extreme excess lower face height (88 mm, UFH:LFH ratio = 0.69), and extreme anterior open bite. The patient had been previously treated orthodontically and was referred for retreatment because the prior treatment had failed. The parents and the patient declined a surgical approach for correction of the malocclusion despite the severe mandibular asymmetry. There was a long history of airway obstruction which had been resolved and the airway was clear at the time of treatment.

relief of severe nasopharyngeal obstruction after adenoidectomy with a subsequent changed breathing mode. There was no orthodontic treatment.

Figure 7-5 and Tables 7-3 and 7-4 illustrate the treatment result of a posterior occlusal bite block and magnetic vertical correctors in patient D.R., a 17-year-old boy with excess lower face height. The figure shows the horizontal expression of mandibular growth that occurred. Expression of the direction and amount of mandibular growth parallel to the functional occlusal plane maximizes the effect of small amounts of mandibular growth in the correction of mandibular retrognathism.

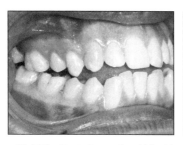
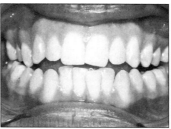
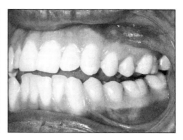

Fig 7-5c Posterior occlusal bite blocks were used to close the bite to the situation illustrated.

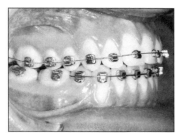
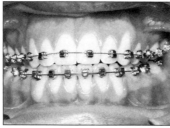
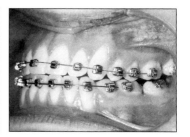

Fig 7-5d Following this, the Class III malocclusion that resulted was corrected with a combination of mandibular premolar extraction and the Speed appliance.

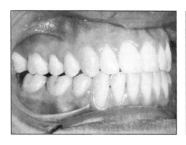
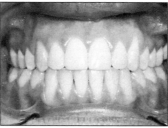
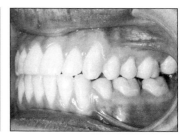

Fig 7-5e Class III malocclusion corrected.

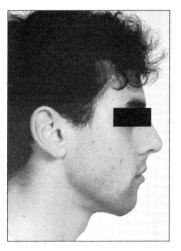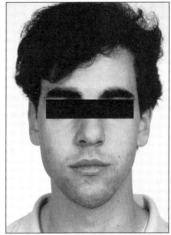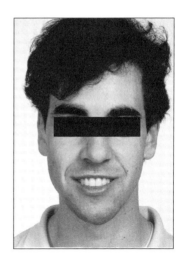

Fig 7-5f Facial photographs of corrected malocclusion.

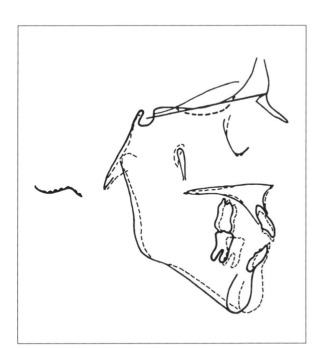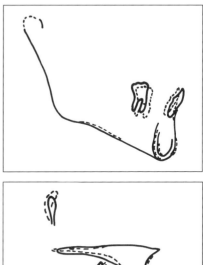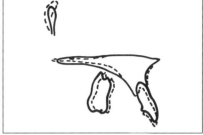

Fig 7-5g The superimposed tracings of patient D.R. show that mandibular length continued to increase. This increased growth, which probably would have been expressed vertically at the chin, was in fact expressed horizontally to produce a relative mandibular autorotation. The tracings also show the small amounts of molar intrusion responsible for the relative mandibular autorotation.

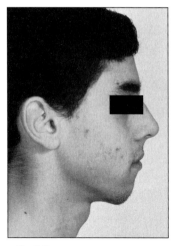 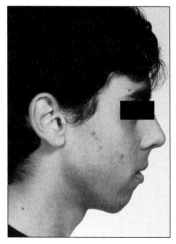 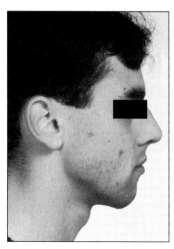

Fig 7-5h The photographs show the serial improvement in facial appearance as treatment progressed.

Cephalometric Identification of Skeletal Dysplasia

The true skeletal pattern of many malocclusions may be camouflaged by either upward and forward or downward and backward vertical mandibular rotations. These rotations occur in response to either a reduction or an increase in alveolar height. A reduction in alveolar height occurs when some neuromuscular factor such as the tongue is postured between the occlusal surfaces of the teeth and inhibits tooth eruption. Overclosure can then occur. Conversely, increased alveolar height occurs when some neuromuscular factor, such as chronic mouth-open mandibular posture, separates the jaws chronically and permits excess alveolar development. Excess lower anterior face height then occurs.

Conventional cephalometric analyses used to measure dysplasia between the jaws will not identify the true skeletal characteristics of such vertical malocclusions. For example, in an overclosed case, a short mandible may be rotated up and forward into an orthognathic position. The SNB angle will indicate an orthognathic mandible in the overclosed position, whereas mandibular retrognathism would be indicated in the rest position. Conversely, if the mandible is rotated down and back into an excess lower face height, the SNB angle might indicate mandibular retrognathism when, in fact, the mandible would be orthognathic in its normal upward and forward position. It thus becomes necessary to use a simple cephalometric analysis that will clearly identify the true skeletal nature of orthodontic problems. Such a simple analysis consists of a triangle formed by the maxillary length, mandibular length, and lower anterior face height (see Fig 1-23).

Class II and Class III malocclusions with dysplasia are difficult to correct by conventional orthodontic treatment when a severe mismatch in size exists between the maxilla and the mandible. The skeletal size matching measurement is used to assess whether the jaws match each other in size within limits that will permit orthodontic correction of the dysplasia. These limits are established by measuring the maxillary and mandibular unit length as illustrated in Fig 1-23. The difference between the two values is called the skeletal size difference. Class II malocclusions characterized by difference values less than 16 mm at age 12 are difficult to manage by conventional orthodontic treatment. Class III dysplasias with unit difference values greater than 29 mm at age 12 are often reserved for either unconventional orthodontic treatment or correction by surgical intervention. The size of the jaws and thus the difference between the jaw sizes will not change when the mandible is rotated either up or down. Therefore, the true skeletal dysplasia will be disclosed in each rotated situation regardless of the retrognathism or prognathism of the mandible. While the difference values are useful in identifying the true dys-

plasia, they will not indicate whether the mismatch has occurred in the maxilla, the mandible, or both bones. The individual unit values for each bone indicates where the abnormality exists. Table 7-5 gives the values for the individual unit sizes and the difference values at different age levels in males and females.

Are the Lower Face Height Dimensions Correct?

When the ANB angle is used to assess the presence of dysplasia as mentioned previously, the values obtained in patients whose jaws are overclosed will be misleading. They will be too small in Class II cases and too great in Class III cases. This is because the excess freeway space allows the mandible to overclose to a more prognathic position than it would normally occupy. Lower face height values can be used to warn the clinician that overclosure may be present. The clinician may then check the freeway space clinically to determine if an excess freeway space is actually present. Lower face height values of less than 60 mm at age 12 usually indicate short lower face height with overclosure. In such Class II cases, the ANB values must be increased several degrees, whereas in Class III cases they may be reduced several degrees to permit a realistic assessment of the degree of dysplasia present. In such problems, an examination of skeletal unit differences in combination with an assess-

Table 7-5 Growth Changes in a Random Group of Children Observed on Standard Cephalometric Profile Radiographs*

Males						Females					
1. Maxillary unit length (TM-ANS[†])											
Age	N	Min	Mean	Max	SD	Age	N	Min	Mean	Max	SD
6	118	76	82	90	3.19	6	89	73	30	89	2.96
9	102	80	87	97	3.43	9	79	78	85	93	3.43
12	96	85	92	101	3.73	12	71	80	90	102	4.07
14	66	88	96	108	4.52	14	49	81	92	104	3.69
16	72	93	100	111	4.17	16	53	86	93	105	3.45

2. Mandibular unit length (TM-Pg)											
Age	N	Min	Mean	Max	SD	Age	N	Min	Mean	Max	SD
6	118	90	99	108	3.85	6	88	88	97	105	3.55
9	102	98	107	117	4.40	9	79	94	105	113	3.88
12	96	102	114	127	4.90	12	71	102	113	124	5.20
14	66	107	121	137	6.05	14	49	104	117	128	4.60
16	72	116	127	139	5.25	16	53	109	119	128	4.44

3. Lower face height (ANS-Gn)											
Age	N	Min	Mean	Max	SD	Age	N	Min	Mean	Max	SD
6	118	52	59	72	3.55	6	88	49	57	65	3.22
9	102	53	62	74	4.25	9	79	50	60	70	3.62
12	96	53	64	76	4.62	12	71	53	62	74	4.36
14	66	56	68	82	5.23	14	49	54	64	72	4.39
16	72	57	71	86	5.73	16	53	55	65	74	4.67

4. Mandibular unit (2) minus maxillary unit (1) (Difference [TM-Pg]–[TM-ANS])											
Age	N	Min	Mean	Max	SD	Age	N	Min	Mean	Max	SD
6	118	10	17	27		6	88	10	17	24	
9	102	13	20	28		9	79	13	20	28	
12	96	12	22	30		12	71	16	23	36	
14	66	14	25	38		14	49	18	26	39	
16	72	17	27	39		16	53	19	26	39	

*Enlargement factor: 9.84%. Longitudinal observations made at ages 6, 9, 12, 14, and 16.[34]

[†]Definitions: TM = Temporomandibular point, a point in the articula fossa on the line from prognathion through the condyle that indicates the maximum length of the mandible; ANS = Anterior nasal spine, a point on the lower curvature of the spine where the vertical thickness is 3 mm; Pg = Pogonion; Gn = Gnathion.

ment of lower anterior face height provides a more accurate assessment of dysplasia than do ANB values.

Conversely, patients whose mandibles have been rotated down and back into more retrognathic positions show excess lower face height values. Class II patients with such mandibular rotation show more severely dysplastic ANB values than would be warranted if the accompanying excess height of the alveolar processes were reduced. The mandible would rotate up and forward to a more orthognathic position. Class III patients with downward and backward mandibular rotation have their mandibular prognathism and Class III malocclusion camouflaged. The true ANB values would be disclosed if the excess alveolar height were reduced and the mandible permitted to rotate up and forward to a more correct lower face height value, but to a more prognathic position. Indeed, many Class III dysplasias are masked and resemble Class I or even Class II malocclusions. The use of skeletal unit matching differences in conjunction with lower face height values often clarifies the true nature of these problems (see Table 7-5).

The Frankfurt mandibular angle is used by many clinicians in the same way as lower face height values. However, lower face height values and ratios are simpler to measure and may be more useful.

Ratio of Upper Anterior Face Height to Lower Anterior Face Height

A measurement of lower anterior face height is frequently insufficient to identify the presence of vertical mandibular rotations because of size differences among individuals. For example, an individual may show a large lower anterior face height. When this is compared to the upper face height, it may be found that the upper dimension is also large and the total vertical dimension is normally proportioned. The use of the ratio of upper face height to lower face height provides a simple method to check such proportionality. Table 5-4 provides ratios for various racial groups. While the standard deviation for these ratios is large (approximately ± 0.05),[47] ratios of .80 at age 12 and older for both sexes serve as useful screening tools. Individuals with ratios of .75 or less usually represent excess lower face height cases. Ratios of .67 or less are often considered to be future surgical cases requiring Le Fort I maxillary impaction to normalize vertical proportions. Conversely, ratios of .85 or greater usually indicate short lower anterior face height cases with overclosure. Table 5-4 gives North American Caucasian population standards (Burlington, Canada; Kings College, England) for anterior face height ratios for both sexes at various ages.

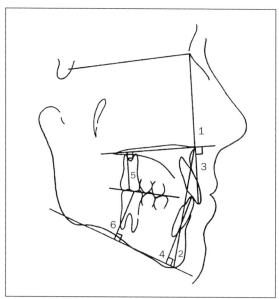

Fig 7-6 Projected measurement for incisor and molar heights in both jaws: 1 = upper anterior face height (N-ANS); 2 = lower anterior face height (ANS-Me); 3 = maxillary incisor height (apical point of maxillary central incisor to palatal plane); 4 = mandibular incisor height (incisal point of mandibular central incisor to mandibular plane); 5 = maxillary molar height (apical point of maxillary first molar to palatal plane); 6 = mandibular molar height (incisal point of mandibular first molar to mandibular plane).

Incisor and Molar Alveolar Height

When the mandible rotates to an inferior position, the molar alveolar height usually increases as the teeth erupt in harmony with the new mandibular position. The incisor alveolar height may also increase depending on the tongue's adaptation to the new mandibular position. If the tongue advances to increase the pharyngeal airway,[59] incisor eruption will be inhibited. The incisors may lose their lingual support and compensate lingually.[57] In other instances, the incisors may supraerupt to an increased alveolar height with an increased display of gingival tissue both at rest and in broad smiling. Such cases will require total arch intrusion at the molar and incisor areas. It is useful to have population standards for vertical dental and alveolar height so that the clinician can clearly identify those areas that require intrusion (Fig 7-6 and Table 7-6).

On the other hand, some deep overbites may be the result of reduced molar height and not increased incisor height. Population standards for molar height would clarify the situation (see Table 7-6).

Table 7-6 Posterior and Anterior Maxillary and Mandibular Heights of Molars and Incisors

	Males (N = 188)		Females (N = 156)	
	Mean	**SD**	**Mean**	**SD**
Maxillary molar height	20.40	2.03	20.58	2.04
Mandibular molar height	28.87	2.12	28.24*	1.92
Maxillary incisor height	28.83	2.51	27.89[†]	2.43
Mandibular incisor height	39.88	2.68	38.83[†]	2.40

(Length in mm)

*P < 0.01
[†] P < 0.001

Burlington Growth Centre (age 12)[47]

Analysis of Anterior Nasopharyngeal Dimensions

Nasopharyngeal airway size is particularly important in determining whether the mode of breathing is nasal or oral. The posterior nasopharyngeal wall is covered by lymphoid tissue that often undergoes hypertrophy during the period prior to puberty. This enlargement of adenoids increases the chance for nasopharyngeal airway obstruction. However, the relationship between the bony nasopharynx size and adenoid size is crucial.[50,74,75,88]

Population standards for the sagittal depth of the bony nasopharynx for males and females are shown in Figs 7-7 and 7-8. There is a steady increase in the sagittal depth of the nasopharynx of males between ages 6 and 20. This increase is on average smaller from ages 6 to 12 (2.4 mm) than from ages 12 to 18 (4.7 mm). The increase in females appears to be negligible after 16 years of age.[102]

In earlier investigations,[51,52] it was found that the sagittal depth of the bony nasopharynx influenced the mode of breathing. In children who were predominantly mouth breathers, the bony nasopharynx was smaller than that found in nose breathers of the same age. Following a change to nose breathing, the bony nasopharynx depth normalized. In addition to the bony changes, a change in the tone of the muscle ring consisting of the orbicularis oris, the buccinator, and the superior pharyngeal constrictor occurred.

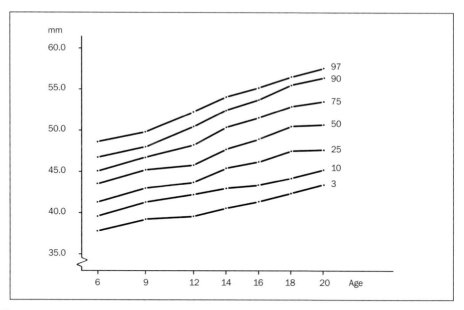

Fig 7-7 Percentile distance curves for sagittal depth of the nasopharynx (Ptm-Ba) for a large sample of males ages 6 through 20 years (Burlington Growth Centre sample).

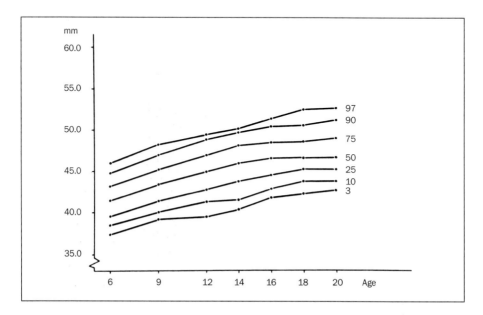

Fig 7-8 Percentile distance curves for sagittal depth of the nasopharynx (Ptm-Ba) for a large sample of females ages 6 through 20 years (Burlington Growth Centre sample).

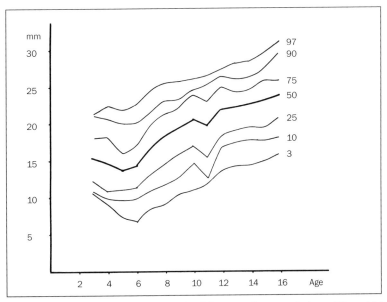

Fig 7-9 Percentile distance curves for the sagittal depth of the nasopharyngeal airway (Ptm-ad$_1$) for boys and girls (Burlington Growth Centre and London King's College samples).

Also, altered muscle tone due to the accompanying change in posture of the head and jaws[75,81] can further reduce the bony airway. The fact that the bony nasopharynx depth normalized following adenoidectomy and the establishment of nose breathing indicates a strong neuromuscular influence in the size of this bony dimension.

There have been few studies of the growth and development of the soft tissues on the posterior nasopharyngeal wall. Tanner,[92] who quoted the classical growth curves of Scammon, stated that the lymphoid tissue of tonsils, adenoids, appendix, intestine, and spleen reaches a maximum volume before adolescence and then declines to the adult state. Handelman and Pruzansky[32] used the lateral cephalometric radiograph to classify the adenoids as sparse, small, medium, or large. They reported that large adenoids were most frequently observed between ages 4 and 6, becoming less frequent in the older groups. There also appeared to be great variation in adenoid size in individuals of similar age.

A reliable indication of the need for otologic examination can be obtained if the clinical record of the mode of breathing can be supplemented by radiocephalometric data on the anteroposterior size of the nasopharyngeal airway. Figure 7-9 shows that, on average, there was a temporary decrease in the sagittal depth of the nasopharyn-

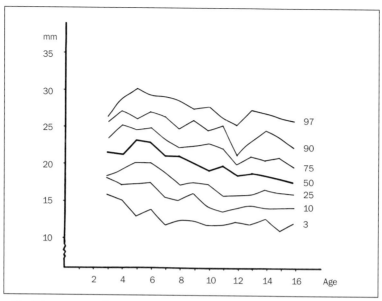

Fig 7-10 Percentile distance curves for the thickness of the soft tissue (ad$_1$-Ba) for boys and girls (Burlington Growth Centre and London King's College samples).

geal airway between ages 3 and 5 and again between ages 10 and 11, with the largest decrease at age 5. Thus the pharyngeal airway is narrowest at age 5. Figure 7-10 shows the thickness of soft tissue on the posterior nasopharyngeal wall (ad$_1$-Ba) along the line joining the posterior nasal spine and basion (Ptm-Ba). The 50th percentile curve shows that this tissue is thickest at age 5, subsequently decreasing to age 16, but with a slight increase at age 11. The course of this curve matches the 50th percentile curve for the size of the nasopharyngeal airway (Ptm-ad$_1$) as shown in Fig 7-9.

The 50th percentile distance curves of the sagittal depth of the airway through the nasopharynx (Ptm-ad$_1$),

the thickness of the soft tissue on the posterior nasopharyngeal wall along the line Ptm-Ba (ad$_1$-Ba), and the sagittal depth of the bony nasopharynx (Ptm-Ba) are compared in Fig 7-11.

Sexual Dimorphism

As can be expected, both the bony nasopharynx and the airway are larger in males (Figs 7-12 and 7-13). However, the adenoid tissue is larger in girls (Fig 7-14). This means that in girls a consistently larger proportion of the pharyngeal space is occupied by the adenoid tissue. We might therefore expect that facial and dental development of girls would be more sensitive to the effects

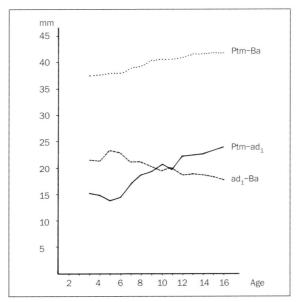

Fig 7-11 Fiftieth percentile distance curves of the sagittal depth of the airway (Ptm-ad$_1$), the thickness of the soft tissue on the posterior nasopharyngeal wall (ad$_1$-Ba), the sagittal depth of the bony nasopharynx (Ptm-Ba) (Burlington Growth Centre and London King's College samples).

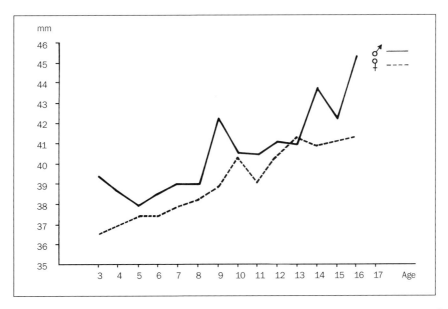

Fig 7-12 Comparison of the skeletal depth of the bony nasopharynx (Ptm-Ba) in males and females (Burlington Growth Centre sample).

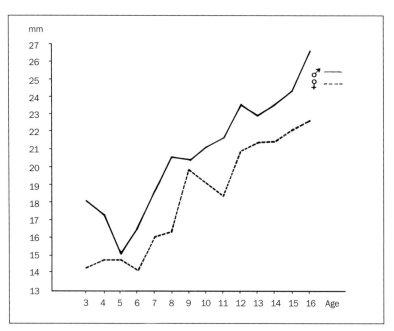

Fig 7-13 Comparison of the depth of the nasopharyngeal airway (Ptm-ad$_1$) in males and females (London King's College sample).

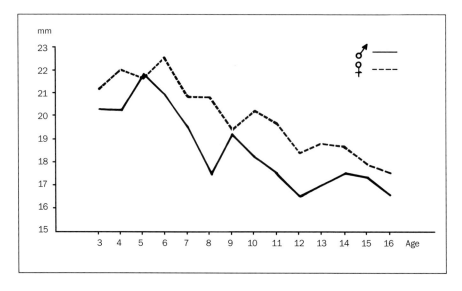

Fig 7-14 Comparison of the adenoid tissue thickness (ad$_1$-Ba) between males and females (London King's College sample).

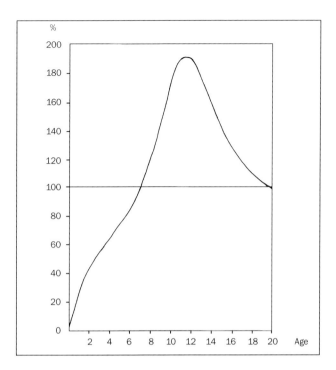

Fig 7-15 Scammon's curve for the growth of the lymphoid tissue of the appendix, spleen, and thymus.

of chronic airway obstruction than boys. This, in fact, is the case.[57] Thus, the growth of the adenoids and of the soft tissues on the nasopharyngeal wall do not follow Scammon's classical lymphatic cycle where the tissues were thought to attain maximum bulk between ages 9 and 15 with subsequent atrophy (Fig 7-15). This classical lymphoid growth curve did not include measurements of the tonsils and adenoids. Scammon's lymphoid growth curve was based on the weight of the thymus, the number of Peyer's patches, the number of lymphoid follicles in the appendix, and the weight of the mesenteric lymphoid tissue. The clinical significance of our findings is obvious. If these tissues do not start to atrophy after ages 5 to 6, the patient may be at risk of developing dentofacial abnormality. It is, therefore, valuable to supplement clinical techniques for establishing the mode of breathing with a simple, objective method for estimating the size of the nasopharyngeal airway.

Since a lateral cephalometric analysis already forms part of the diagnostic routine in most orthodontic cases, it is often chosen for the assessment. Because the nasopharyngeal space increases with the age of the child and

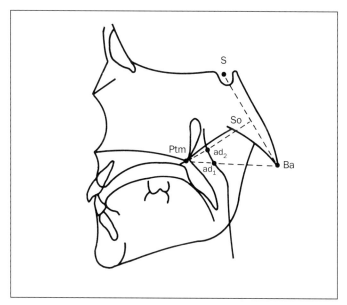

Fig 7-16 Reference points: Ptm = pterygomaxillary; S = sella turcica; Ba = basion; So = the midpoint on the line joining S and Ba; ad_1 = the intersection of the posterior nasopharyngeal wall and the line Ptm-Ba; ad_2 = the intersection of the posterior nasopharyngeal wall and the line Ptm-So. These measurements give the size of the airway at two different levels.

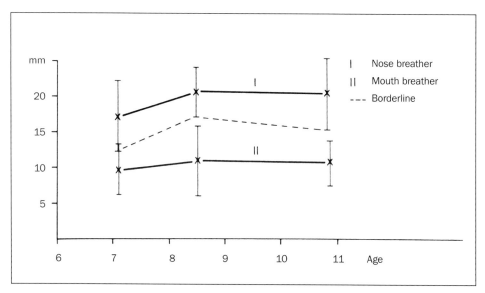

Fig 7-17 Diagram of means and SD for airway size (Ptm-ad_1) for 54 mouth breathers and 55 nose breathers ages 6 through 11 (Örebro sample). These measurements give the size of the airway at two different levels.

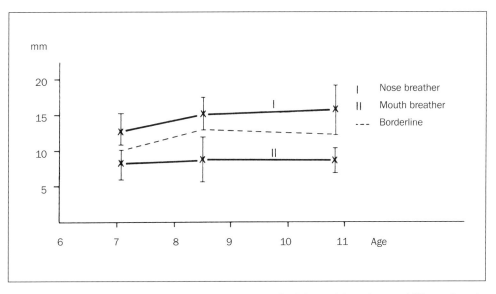

Fig 7-18 Diagram of means and SD for airway size (Ptm-ad$_2$) for 54 mouth breathers and 55 nose breathers ages 6 through 11 (Örebro sample).

the lymphoid tissue on the posterior wall of the nasopharynx usually diminishes before puberty, it is helpful to have standards for the sagittal size of the nasopharyngeal airway at different ages. It must be fully recognized that we are actually dealing with a three-dimensional space that is seen in only two dimensions on the radiograph. Such standards are provided for children ages 6 through 11 because these are the ages usually involved in orthodontic treatment. The cephalometric analysis of the lateral radiographs has only two reference points (ad$_1$ and ad$_2$) on the posterior wall of the nasopharynx added to accomplish the

desired assessment. Measurements of the distances Ptm-ad$_1$ and Ptm-ad$_2$ (Fig 7-16) give a good indication of the anteroposterior size of the nasopharyngeal airway. Current practice should be followed for clinical registration of mode of breathing. An otologic examination of the nasopharynx is recommended in cases where the measured distance Ptm-ad$_1$ or Ptm-ad$_2$ is less than the mean minus 1 standard deviation for nose breathers in the corresponding age group. The patients should also complain of obstructed breathing. The boundary is marked with a broken line in Figs 7-17 and 7-18.[53]

Summary

An appreciation of craniofacial variation in the vertical dimension should play a prominent role in any orthodontic clinician's approach to the diagnosis and treatment of malocclusion. Our previous investigations show that malocclusions characterized by excess lower face height occur in approximately 18% of Caucasian males, whereas 26% have short lower face height.[56,102] It is probable that these percentages accumulate at a higher level in orthodontic practices.

Study of the vertical dimension provides an excellent model to support the view that many malocclusions previously thought to be of genetic origin are, in reality, neuromuscular imitations of genetically based problems. This is an important concept because if it is true, it implies that such malocclusion could be partially reversed by removal of the neuromuscular impact. An example of such removal would be the change from chronic mouth breathing to nose breathing. Our previous work has shown a horizontal expression of mandibular growth direction without orthodontic treatment following a change in the patient's biologic status as in the earlier example.[58] We have also shown normalization of mandibular incisor inclination from lingually to more labially inclined incisors without orthodontic treatment. This followed a biologic change such as changed mode of breathing.[57,104] Our assumption is that large changes in skeletal and dental patterns of malocclusion, previously thought to be genetic, can be accomplished when biologic correction accompanies orthodontic therapy of vertical malocclusions.

There has been considerable debate about the stability of orthodontic treatment during recent years. Most of this debate has centered around mandibular incisor alignment. Our work shows clearly that an important factor in assisting stability of incisor alignment would be a reversal in the development of excess lower face height through the establishment of mouth-closed breathing.

Since vertical relationships seem to deteriorate progressively with time in cases with chronic nasopharyngeal obstruction,[102] it would seem logical to interfere biologically as early as possible in those individuals who show altered mandibular posture in association with such obstruction. Since the deterioration is progressive up to maturity, it might never be too late to attempt some improvement in adolescents.

In summary, the neuromuscular suspension of the mandible is a highly sensitive mechanism that responds with altered mandibular posture in some cases of chronic nasopharyngeal obstruction. When this alteration occurs, associated changes such as increased lower face height, mandibular retrognathism, narrow arches, and incisor crowding accompany the primary change to various degrees in individual patients.[50,57,103-105] Treatment of excess face height malocclusions is one of the more challenging areas of orthodontic treatment. The large variability in an individual's response to similar adverse environmental stimuli complicates clinical management.

References

1. Adamidis IP, Spyropoulos MN. The effects of lymphadenoid hypertrophy on the position of the tongue, the mandible and the hyoid bone. Eur J Orthod 1983;5:287–294.

2. Ågren K, Nordlander B, Linder-Aronson S, Zettergren-Wijk L, Svanborg E. Children with nocturnal upper airway obstruction: Postoperative orthodontic and respiratory improvement. Acta Otolaryngol 1998;118: 581–587.

3. Alexander TL, Hitchcock HP. Cephalometric standards for American Negro children. Am J Orthod 1978;74:298–304.

4. Altemus LA. A comparison of cephalofacial relationships. Angle Orthod 1960;30:223–240.

5. Altuna G, Woodside DG. Die Auswirkung von Ausbissblock im Oberkiefer bei Macaca rhesus. Fortschr Kieferorthop 1977;4:391–403.

6. Altuna G, Woodside DG. The relationship between lower face height and inclination of the incisor [abstract 947]. J Dent Res 1989; 68:300.

7. Andersson L, Brattström V. Cephalometric analysis of permanently snoring patients with and without obstructive sleep apnea syndrome. Int J Oral Maxillofac Surg 1991;20:159–162.

8. Archer SY, Vig PS. Effects of head position on intraoral pressures in Class I and Class II adults. Am J Orthod 1985;87:311–318.

9. Behlfelt K. Enlarged tonsils and the effect of tonsillectomy. Characteristics of the dentition and facial skeleton. Posture of the head, hyoid bone and tongue. Mode of breathing. Swed Dent J Suppl 1990;72:1–35.

10. Behlfelt K, Linder-Aronson S. Große Tonsillen und deren Einfluß auf die Kopf und Zungenhaltung. Fortschr Kieferorthop 1988;49:476–483.

11. Bhatia SN, Leighton BC. A Manual of Facial Growth: A Computer Analysis of Longitudinal Cephalometric Growth Data. New York: Oxford Univ Press, 1993.

12. Brash JC, McKeag HTA, Scott JH. The Aetiology of Irregularity and Malocclusion of Teeth. London: Dental Board of the United Kingdom, 1956.

13. Bresolin D, Shapiro PA, Shapiro GG, Chapko MK, Dassel S. Mouth breathing in allergic children: Its relationship to dentofacial development. Am J Orthod 1983; 83:334–340.

14. Burlington Orthodontic Research Centre Progress Report Series 1, 2, 3, 4. Burlington Growth Centre, Faculty of Dentistry, Univ of Toronto, 1954–1957.

15. Bushey RS. Alterations in certain anatomical relations accompanying the change from oral to nasal breathing [thesis]. Univ of Illinois, 1965.

16. Bushey RS. Recent research findings relating nasopharyngeal function to oral physiology and craniofacial development. Proc Found Orthod Res 1973:17-63.

17. Cartwright LJ, Harvold EP. Improved radiographic results in cephalometry through the use of high kilovoltage. J Can Dent Assoc 1954;20:261–263.

18. Cole P. Respiratory rhinometry: A review of recent trends. Rhinology 1980;18:3–8.

19. Cole P. Nose, upper airway physiology and the atmospheric environment. In: Proctor DF, Andersen IB (eds). New York: Elsevier Biomedical Press, 1982:164–189.

20. Cole P, Fastag O, Niinimaa V. Computer-aided rhinometry: A research rhinometer for clinical trial. Acta Otolaryngol 1980; 90:139–142.

21. Cole P, Havas T. Resistance to respiratory airflow of the nasal passages: Comparisons between different common methods of calculation. Rhinology 1986;24:163–173.

22. Cotton WN, Takano WS, Wong WMW. The Downs analysis applied to three other ethnic groups. Angle Orthod 1951;21:213–220.

23. Davies PL. Electromyographic study of superficial neck muscles in mandibular function. J Dent Res 1979;58:537–538.

24. De Montbeillard PG, Scammon RE. The first seratim study of human growth. Am J Phys Anthropol 1927;10:329–336.

25. Dunn GF, Green LJ, Cunat JJ. Relationships between variation of mandibular morphology and variation of nasopharyngeal airway size in monozygotic twins. Angle Orthod 1973;43:129–135.

26. Eckhardt PG, Bijlmer RP. Obstructive sleep apnea syndrome. Tijdschr Kindergeneeskd 1984;52:212.

27. Fränkel R, Fränkel C. Orofacial Orthopedics with the Function Regulator. Basel: Karger 1989.

28. Freng A. Congenital choanal atresia. Etiology, morphology and diagnosis in 82 cases. Scand J Plast Reconstr Surg 1978;12:261–265.

29. Freng A. Dentofacial development in long-lasting nasal stenosis. Scand J Dent Res 1979;87:260–267.

30. Freng A, Kvam E. Facial sagittal growth following partial basal resection of the nasal septum: A retrospective study in man. Eur J Orthod 1979;1:89–96.

31. Graamans K. The significance of nasal resistance under normal and pathological conditions. Acta Otorhinolaryngol Belg 1979; 33:495–499.

32. Handelman CS, Pruzansky S. The size of the adenoids in normal and C.P.I. children. Presented at the IADR, Washington, DC, 1967.

33. Hannuksela A. The effect of moderate and severe atophy on the facial skeleton. Eur J Orthod 1981;3:187–193.

34. Harvold EP. Some biological aspects of orthodontic treatment in the transitional dentition. Am J Orthod 1963;49:1–14.

35. Harvold EP. The role of function in the etiology and treatment of malocclusion. Am J Orthod 1968;54:883–898.

36. Harvold EP. The Activator in Interceptive Orthodontics. St Louis: Mosby, 1974.

37. Harvold EP. Neuromuscular and morphological adaptations in experimentally induced oral respiration. In: McNamara JA (ed). Nasorespiratory Function and Craniofacial Growth, monograph 9. Craniofacial Growth Series. Ann Arbor, MI: Univ of Michigan 1979:149–164.

38. Harvold EP. Treatment of Hemifacial Microsomia. New York: Alan R. Liss, 1983.

39. Harvold EP, Chierici G, Vargervik K. Experiments on the development of dental malocclusions. Am J Orthod 1972;61:38–44.

40. Harvold EP, Poyton HG. Syndrome of dual bite associated with open bite. J Can Dent Assoc 1962;28:617–626.

41. Harvold EP, Tomer BS, Vargervik K, Chierici G. Primate experiments on oral respiration. Am J Orthod 1981; 79:359–372.

42. Hellsing E. Changes in the pharyngeal airway in relation to extension of the head. Eur J Orthod 1989;11:359–365.

43. Hellsing E, L'Estrange P. Changes in lip pressure following extension and flexion of the head and at changed mode of breathing. Am J Orthod Dentofacial Orthop 1987;91:286–294.

44. Hellsing E, Forsberg C-M, Linder-Aronson S, Sheikholeslam A. Changes in postural EMG activity in the neck and masticatory muscles following obstruction of the nasal airways. Eur J Orthod 1986;8:247–253.

45. Holik R. Relation between habitual breathing through the mouth and muscular activity of the tongue. Ceska Stomatol 1957;57:170.

46. Hultcrantz E, Larson M, Hellquist R, Ahlquist-Rastad J, Svanholm H, Jakobsson OP. The influence of tonsillar obstruction and tonsillectomy on facial growth and dental arch morphology. Int J Pediatr Otorhinolaryngol 1991; 22:125–134.

47. Janson GR, Metaxas A, Woodside DG. Variation in maxillary and mandibular molar and incisor vertical dimension in 12 year old subjects with excess, normal and short lower anterior face height. Am J Orthod Dentofacial Orthop 1994;106:409–418.

48. Kern EB. Standardization of rhinomanometry. Rhinology 1977;15:115–119.

49. Larsson E. Dummy- and fingersucking habits with special attention to their significance for facial growth and occlusion. Tandläkartidningen 1973; 65:1039–1042.

50. Linder-Aronson S. Adenoids: Their effect on mode of breathing and nasal airflow and their relationship to characteristics of the facial skeleton and the dentition. A biometric, rhino-manometric and cephalometro-radiographic study on children with and without adenoids [thesis]. Acta Otolaryngol Suppl 1970;265:1-132.

51. Linder-Aronson S. Effects of adenoidectomy on dentition and nasopharynx. Trans Eur Orthod Soc 1972;177–186.

52. Linder-Aronson S. Effects of adenoidectomy on the dentition and facial skeleton over a period of five years. In: Cook JT (ed). Transactions of the Third International Orthodontic Congress. London: Crosby Lockwood Staples, 1975:85–100.

53. Linder-Aronson S, Henrikson CO. Radio-cephalometric analysis of anteroposterior nasopharyngeal dimensions in 6 to 12-year old mouth breathers compared with nose breathers. ORL J Otorhinolaryngol Relat Spec 1973; 35:19–29.

54. Linder-Aronson S, Woodside DG, Daigle DJ. A longitudinal study of the growth in length of the maxilla in boys between ages 6-20 years. Trans Eur Orthod Soc 1975;169-179.

55. Linder-Aronson S, Leighton BC. A longitudinal study of the development of the posterior nasopharyngeal wall between 3 and 16 years of age. Eur J Orthod 1983;5:47–58.

56. Linder-Aronson S, Woodside DG. Some craniofacial variables related to small or diminishing lower anterior face height. Swed Dent J Suppl 1982;15:131–146.

57. Linder-Aronson S, Woodside DG, Hellsing E, Emerson W. Normalization of incisor position after adenoidectomy. Am J Orthod Dentofacial Orthop 1993;103:412–427.

58. Linder-Aronson S, Woodside DG, Lundstrom A. Mandibular growth direction following adenoidectomy. Am J Orthod 1986;89:273–284.

59. Lowe A. Correlations between orofacial muscle activity and craniofacial morphology in a sample of control and anterior open bite subjects. Am J Orthod 1980;78:89–98.

60. Lowe AA, Gionhaku N, Takeuchi K, Fleetham JA. Three-dimensional CT reconstructions of tongue and airway in adult subjects with obstructive sleep apnea. Am J Orthod Dentofacial Orthop 1986;90:364–374.

61. Lundström A, McWilliam JS. A comparison of vertical and horizontal cephalometric variables with regard to heritability. Eur J Orthod 1987;9:104–108.

62. Lundström A, Woodside DG. Individual variation in growth directions expressed at the chin and the midface. Eur J Orthod 1980;2:65–79.

63. Masaki F. The longitudinal study of morphological differences in the cranial base and facial structure between Japanese and American whites. J Jpn Orthod Soc 1980; 39:436–456.

64. McNamara JA. Experimental examination of growth of the lower jaw [German]. Inf Orthod Kieferorthop 1976;8:219–243.

65. McNamara JA, Jr. An experimental study of increased vertical dimension in the growing face. Am J Orthod 1977;71:382–395.

66. Miura F, Soma K, Kuroki T. An Atlas of Dento-Craniofacial Morphology of Peruvian and Mexican Indians. First Department of Orthodontics, Faculty of Dentistry, Tokyo Medical and Dental Univ, 1995.

67. Niinimaa V, Cole P, Mintz S, Shephard RJ. Head-out exercise body plethysmograph. J Appl Physiol 1979; 47:1336–1339.

68. Parker LP. Diagnostic rhinomanometry using "headout" volume displacement plethysmography on 1,000 consecutive subjects [thesis]. Toronto: Univ of Toronto, 1987.

69. Parker LP, Crysdale WS, Cole P, Woodside DG. Rhinomanometry in children. Int J Pediatr Otorhinolaryngol 1989;17:127–137.

70. Persson M, Sundell S. Facial morphology and open bite deformity in amelogenesis imperfecta. A roentgenocephalometric study. Acta Odontol Scand 1982;40:135–144.

71. Peterson DS. Progressive nasal obstruction: Head position and head posture [thesis]. Toronto: Univ of Toronto, 1990.

72. Petri N, Suadicani P, Wildschiodtz G, Bjorn-Jorgensen J. Predictive value of Muller maneuver, cephalometry and clinical features for the outcome of uvulopalatopharyngoplasty. Evaluation of predictive factors using discriminant analysis in 30 sleep apnea patients. Acta Otolaryngol 1994;114:565–571.

73. Richardson ER. Atlas of Craniofacial Growth in Americans of African Descent. Ann Arbor, MI: Univ of Michigan, 1980.

74. Ricketts RM. The cranial base and soft structures in cleft palate speech and breathing. Plast Reconstr Surg 1954;14:47.

75. Ricketts RM. Respiratory obstructions and their relation to tongue posture. Cleft Palate Bull 1958;8:4–5.

76. Ricketts RM. Respiratory obstruction syndrome. Am J Orthod 1968; 54:495–507.

77. Riolo ML. An Atlas of Craniofacial Growth. Ann Arbor, MI: Univ of Michigan, 1974.

78. Sakamoto T, Miura F, Iizuka T. Linear analysis on the development changes of dentofacial complex of Japanese by means of roentgenographic cephalometry. J Jpn Stomat Soc 1963;30:169–207.

79. Solow B, Greve E. Craniocervical angulation and nasal respiratory resistance in naso-respiratory function and craniofacial growth. In: McNamara JA (ed). Nasorespiratory Function and Craniofacial Growth, monograph 9. Craniofacial Growth Series. Ann Arbor, MI: Univ of Michigan, 1979:87-119.

80. Solow B, Greve E. Rhinomanometric recording in children. Rhinology 1980;18:31–42.

81. Solow B, Kreiborg S. Soft-tissue stretching: A possible control factor in craniofacial morphogenesis. Scand J Dent Res 1977;85: 505–507.

82. Solow B, Ovesen J, Nielsen PW, Wildschiodtz G, Tallgren A. Head posture in obstructive sleep apnoea. Eur J Orthod 1993;15:107–114.

83. Solow B, Siersbaek-Nielsen S, Greve E. Airway adequacy, head postures and craniofacial morphology. Am J Orthod 1984;86: 214–223.

84. Solow B, Skov S, Ovesen J, Norup P, Wildschiodtz G. Airway dimensions and head posture in obstructive sleep apnoea. Eur J Orthod 1996;18:571–579.

85. Solow B, Sonnesen L. Head posture and malocclusions. Eur J Orthod 1998; 20:685–693.

86. Solow B, Tallgren A. Head posture and craniofacial morphology. Am J Phys Anthropol 1976;44:417–435.

87. Spyropolous MN. An early approach for the interception of skeletal open bite: A preliminary report. J Pedod 1985;9:200–209.

88. Subtelny JD. The significance of adenoid tissue in orthodontia. Angle Orthod 1954; 24:59–69.

89. Subtelny JD. A cephalometric study of the growth of the soft palate. Plast Reconstr Surg 1957;19:49–62.

90. Subtelny JD, Nieto RPP. A longitudinal study of maxillary growth following pharyngeal flap surgery. Cleft Palate J 1978;15:118–131.

91. Takahashi S, Ono T, Ishiwata Y, Kuroda T. Effect of changes in the breathing mode and body position on tongue pressure with respiratory-related oscillations. Am J Orthod Dentofacial Orthop 1999;115:239–246.

92. Tanner JM. The human growth curve. In: Harrison GA, Weiner JS, Tanner JM, Barnicot NA (eds). Human Biology. New York: Oxford Univ Press, 1964:310.

93. Tanner JM, Whitehouse RH, Takaishi M. Standards from birth to maturity for height, weight, height velocity and weight velocity: British children, 1965. I Arch Dis Child 1966;41:454–471.

94. Thompson D. Growth and Form, vol 1. Cambridge: The University Press, 1959.

95. Tourne LPM. The long face syndrome and impairment of the nasopharyngeal airway. Angle Orthod 1990;60:167–176.

96. Vig SP. Respiration, nasal airway and orthodontics: A review of current clinical concepts and research. In: Johnston LE (ed). New Vistas in Orthodontics. Philadelphia: Lea & Febeiger, 1985.

97. Vig SP, Showfety KJ, Phillips C. Experimental manipulation of head posture. Am J Orthod 1980;77:258–268.

98. Wenzel A, Henriksen J, Melsen B. Nasal respiratory resistance and head posture: Effect of intranasal corticosteroid (Budesonide) in children with asthma and perennial rhinitis. Am J Orthod 1983;84:422–426.

99. Woodside DG. Distance, velocity and relative growth rate standards for mandibular growth for Caucasian males and females aged three to twenty years [thesis]. St. Louis, MO: American Board of Orthodontics, 1971.

100. Woodside DG. A serial study of mandibular growth accelerations in a large population of Caucasian males and females aged three to twenty years. In: Hosl E, Baldaulf A (eds). Mechanical and Biological Basics in Orthodontic Therapy. Heidelberg: Herthig, 1991.

101. Woodside DG, Altuna G, Harvold E, Herbert M, Metaxas A. Primate experiments in malocclusion and bone induction. Am J Orthod 1983; 83:460–468.

102. Woodside DG, Linder-Aronson S. The channelization of upper and lower anterior face heights compared to population standard in males between ages 6 to 20 years. Eur J Orthod 1979;1:25–40.

103. Woodside DG, Linder-Aronson S. Progressive increase in lower anterior face height and the use of the posterior occlusal bite blocks and its management. In: Graber L (ed). Orthodontics: State of the Art, Essence of the Science. St Louis: Mosby, 1986:200–211.

104. Woodside DG, Linder-Aronson S, Lundström A, McWilliam J. Mandibular and maxillary growth after changed mode of breathing. Am J Orthod Dentofacial Orthop 1991; 100: 1–18.

105. Woodside DG, Linder-Aronson S, Stubbs DO. Relationship between mandibular incisor crowding and nasal mucosal swelling. Proc Finn Den Soc 1991; 87:127–138.

106. Yip ASG, Cleall JF. Cinefluographic study of velarpharyngeal function before and after removal of tonsils and adenoids. Angle Orthod 1971;41:251.

107. Zeng X, Forsberg C-M, Linder-Aronson S. Craniofacial morphology in Chinese and Swedish children with Class I and Class II relation. Aust Orthod J 1998;15:168–176.

108. Zwaardemaker H. Ademannslag als diagnosticum der nasale stenose. Ned Tijdschr Geneeskd 1889;25:297–300. Cited by: Clement and Hirsch 1984.

Index